<u>*Learn Art Of Intimacy*</u>

"Sex is an art to satisfy your partner "

SexDucation
Key To Satisfy

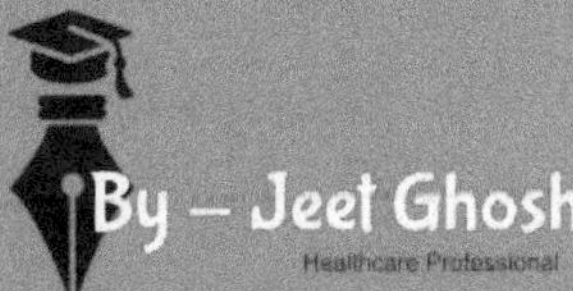

By — Jeet Ghosh
Healthcare Professional

Available On

1st Edition

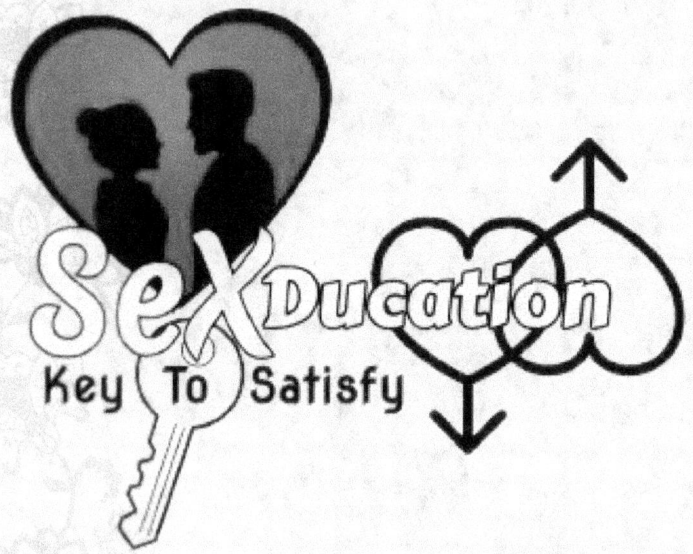

Learn Art Of Intimacy

"Sex is an art to satisfy your partner "

By Mr. Jeet Ghosh

Bsc.Medical Technology (Radiography &Imaging) and DRD (Tech.)
Medical Technologist (Radiodiagnostic) & Healthcare Resource Person

Published in 2024 | India | West Bengal

Preface

"Sexducation : Key to satisfy" is a comprehensive guide that aims to transform your understanding and experience of intimate relationships. This book covers a wide range of topics essential for a fulfilling sexual life, including foundational sex education, the art of intimacy, and the importance of effective sexual communication. It delves into the use of various sexual devices and materials, offering practical advice on how to incorporate them into your intimate moments. Additionally, "Sexducation" provides detailed and sensitive guidance on oral and anal sex, helping you to approach these practices with confidence and care. The book also explores different types of condoms, explaining their uses and benefits to ensure safe and enjoyable experiences.

To further enhance your intimate life, "Sexducation" presents a diverse array of sex positions and offers tips and techniques designed to maximize pleasure and satisfaction for you and your partner. Whether you are looking to deepen your connection, explore new dimensions of intimacy, or simply improve your sexual knowledge, this book is an invaluable resource for anyone seeking to enhance their sexual well-being.

Key Features Of This Book

- Clear And Accessible Language.
- Easy To Understand
- Easy To Remember
- To The Point Discussion
- Concise And Focused Content
- Reader-Friendly Format
- Content Unique Topics "Advance Topics"
- Learn and apply easily

Key Outcome Of This Book

- Enhanced sexual knowledge.
- Understanding your partner's sexual needs
- Learn tricks & techniques to Foreplay
- Learn sexual erogenous zones
- Learn art intimacy to satisfy
- Learn Sex timing Vs sex satisfaction
- Better sexual communication.
- Informed use of sexual devices & material
- Confidence in oral and anal sex to increase pleasure
- Understanding condom types,uses & application
- Variety in sex positions to satisfy
- Techniques for mutual satisfaction
- Tricks to increase sexual pleasure
- Techniques to satisfy your partner
- Learn virtual distance sex

About The Author

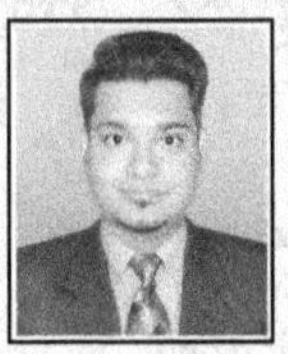

Jeet Ghosh is an experienced medical technologist (Radiography & imaging) having experience of many years in the field of radiography and Imaging. He was a student of Kendriya Vidyalaya and completed a degree in Medical Technology (Radiography and Imaging) from SRHU(Swami Rama Himalayan University) ,HIMS, Jollygrant, Dehradun, Uttrakhand as well as Diploma In Radiography (Diagnostic Tech.) From SMFWB (State Medical Faculty Of West Bengal), Peerless Hospitex Hospital And Research Centre pvt.ltd . He was awarded a distinction, gold medal,merit certificate and nemontonnos for his accademic brilliance in this field.

Worked in various hospitals from uni-speciality to multi-speciality hospitals (corporate/government/semi-govt.) ,from 300 to 1200 beded teaching and non teaching hospitals .Worked in various healthcare training institute as a trainer, faculty and healthcare resource person .

He had trained many students in various domains of healthcare , develops their skills, helping them to establish in the field of healthcare.

He is running a YouTube channel and Facebook page named as "Radtech knowledges with Jeet Ghosh" where various learning long videos & short videos related to Radiography, medical physics and Imaging are available.Link-https://youtube.com   @RadtechKnowledgesWithJeetGhosh   & https://www.facebook.com/RadtechKnowledgesWithJeetGhosh

His skill sets are teaching , written, reading, public speaking, learning content development, Digital learning videos creations,subjective content writing, editing, academic administration, student councilling ,soft digital marketing and performing radiological examinations (X-Ray/CT Scan/MRI)

He believes in the philosophies of Swami Vivekananda

"ज्ञानमेव परमं बलं यद् बलं परमं ज्ञानम्।
विद्यादविनयमेव तत् सर्वभूतेषु व्यवस्थितम्॥"

Which means "Knowledge alone is the supreme strength; supreme strength is knowledge alone.
It is through education and humility that it is established in all beings."

Copyright Notice

https://youtube.com/@RadtechKnowledgesWithJeetGhosh

https://www.facebook.com/@RadtechKnowledgesWithJeetGhosh

SUBSCRIBE
LIKE
SHARE
FOLLOW

Context

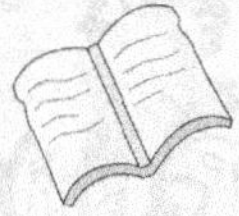 **Chapter Outline** 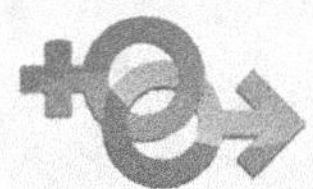

- Communication in sexual Relationships
- Why Communication Matters
- Overcoming sexual communication barrier

- Key sexual Communication Skills
- Effective Communicating About Sex
- Benifit of effective sex

★ ***Communication in Sexual Relationships:***
The Foundation of Sexual Satisfaction

Effective communication is the cornerstone of a healthy and fulfilling relationship. When it comes to sexual satisfaction, communication is vital. In this chapter, we'll delve into the importance of communication in relationships, explore the benefits, and provide practical tips on how to communicate effectively with your partner.

★ ***Why Sexual Communication Matters*** ?

Builds Trust and Understanding :

Communication helps you understand each other's values, beliefs, and desires, fostering a deeper trust and connection. When you communicate openly, you build a foundation of trust, which is essential for a healthy and fulfilling sexual relationship.

Example: Share your thoughts on what intimacy means to you and listen to your partner's perspective.

- ***Prevents Misunderstandings and Conflicts :*** Open communication can prevent miscommunications and conflicts, creating a more harmonious relationship.

  Example: Clarify your expectations and desires to avoid assumptions and potential conflicts.

- ***Helps Understand Each Other's Needs and Desires*** : Communication enables you to understand each other's sexual needs, desires, and boundaries.

  Example: Discuss your love language and how it relates to sexual intimacy.

- ***Creates a Sense of Safety and Security :*** Effective communication creates a safe and supportive environment, allowing you to feel comfortable sharing your thoughts and feelings.

  Example: Establish a "safe word" to stop any uncomfortable sexual activity.

- ***Enhances Emotional Intimacy :*** Communication strengthens emotional intimacy, leading to a more fulfilling and satisfying relationship.

  Example: Practice vulnerability by sharing your fears, desires, and hopes with each other.

★ <u>*Key Sexual Communication Skills*</u>

- **Active Listening :** Give your undivided attention, maintain eye contact, and ask clarifying questions to ensure understanding.

Example: Repeat back what you heard to ensure understanding and show you value your partner's thoughts. Ask open-ended questions to encourage more sharing.

- **Expressing Yourself Clearly and Respectfully :** Share your thoughts, feelings, and desires in a clear and respectful manner. Avoid blaming or attacking language, which can lead to defensiveness and hurt feelings.

Example: Use "I" statements instead of "you" statements, which can come across as accusatory. Instead of "You always ignore my needs," say "I feel neglected when my needs aren't considered."

- **Asking Open-Ended Questions :** Encourage meaningful conversations by asking open-ended questions that begin with what, how, or why. Avoid leading questions or ones that can be answered with a simple "yes" or "no."

Example: Ask "What does intimacy mean to you?" instead of "Do you like intimacy?" This encourages a more in-depth conversation about your partner's desires and needs.

- **Non-Judgmental Feedback :** Provide feedback that is constructive, specific, and free from judgment. Feedback should aim to improve communication and understanding, not criticize or blame.

Example: Focus on the behavior rather than attacking your partner personally. Instead of "You're always late," say "I feel frustrated when we don't leave on time. Can we work on being more punctual?"

- **Emotional Awareness and Empathy :** Be aware of your emotions and empathize with your partner's feelings. Recognize your emotional triggers and acknowledge your partner's emotions.

Example: Recognize your emotional triggers and acknowledge your partner's emotions. If you feel defensive when your partner brings up a sensitive topic, take a step back and acknowledge their feelings before responding.

By cultivating effective communication skills and creating a supportive environment, you'll be better equipped to navigate the complexities of sexual satisfaction in your relationship.

★ *Effective communication in sexual relationship*

- **Discussing Sexual Desires and Preferences :**
communicating with your partner about what you like and dislike in bed, including your sexual desires and preferences. This can include discussing specific acts, positions, and techniques, as well as sharing your fantasies and desires.

Example: Sarah and Mike have a conversation about their sexual desires and preferences. Sarah shares that she loves being touched gently on her neck and back, while Mike reveals that he enjoys exploring new positions. This conversation helps them understand each other's desires and boundaries, making their sexual encounters more enjoyable and fulfilling.

- **Exploring New Sexual Experiences:**This point involves communicating with your partner about trying new things in the bedroom, such as new positions, toys, or role-playing. This can help keep the spark alive in your relationship and prevent boredom.

Example: Emily and Jack have a conversation about trying new things in bed. They discuss their boundaries and what makes them feel uncomfortable, and then try out some new experiences together.

- **Communicating During Sex:** This point involves communicating with your partner during sexual activity, such as telling them what feels good or what you want them to do differently. This can help ensure that both partners are enjoying themselves and can help prevent discomfort or pain.

Example: Rachel and Chris are in the middle of a passionate encounter when Rachel suddenly feels uncomfortable. She communicates her feelings to Chris, who immediately stops and asks what's wrong. They have a quick conversation about what's not feeling right, and then adjust their position to make Rachel more comfortable.

- **Giving and Receiving Feedback:** Giving and receiving feedback involves sharing thoughts and feelings about your sexual experiences with your partner. This can help you understand what works and what doesn't, and can lead to greater sexual satisfaction.

Example: After having sex, David asks his partner, "How was that for you? Was there anything you particularly enjoyed or didn't enjoy?" His partner shares her thoughts, and David listens attentively, using the feedback to adjust his approach for their next encounter.

- **Showing Affection and Intimacy Outside of Sex:**Showing affection and intimacy outside of sex involves displaying physical affection and emotional connection in everyday moments, not just during sexual activity. This can strengthen your bond and create a sense of closeness.

Example: On a Sunday morning, Emily and her partner, Jack, cuddle on the couch, watching a movie together. They hold hands, and Emily rests her head on Jack's shoulder, feeling comfortable and connected.

- **Discussing Sexual Health and Wellness:** Discussing sexual health and wellness involves talking openly about your sexual health, any concerns or issues you have, and your boundaries and preferences. This can help you prioritize your physical and emotional well-being.

Example: Mark and his partner, Laura, have a conversation about their sexual health, discussing their STI status, birth control methods, and any concerns they have. They feel comfortable sharing this information with each other and are grateful for the open communication.

- **Sharing Sexual Fantasies and Desires:** Sharing sexual fantasies and desires involves communicating your deepest desires and fantasies with your partner. This can help you understand each other's needs and boundaries.

Example: Samantha and her partner, Michael, share their sexual fantasies with each other, revealing their deepest desires. They listen without judgment and explore ways to fulfill each other's fantasies.

- **Creating a Safe and Comfortable Environment for Sex:** Creating a safe and comfortable environment for sex involves setting the mood and creating a space where you both feel relaxed and comfortable. This can help you feel more at ease and enjoy the experience more.

Example: James and his partner, Leah, set the mood for a romantic evening, dimming the lights and playing soft music. They create a safe space for each other to feel comfortable and relaxed, making their sexual encounter more enjoyable.

★ *<u>Overcoming Sexual Communication Barriers</u>*

- **Identifying and Challenging Negative Thought Patterns:**Recognize and challenge negative thoughts and beliefs that can lead to communication barriers.

  Example: Sarah notices she often assumes the worst when her partner is late, leading to negative thoughts and feelings. She challenges these thoughts by reminding herself that her partner is responsible and may have a valid reason for being late.

- **Practicing Empathy and Understanding:** Put yourself in your partner's shoes and try to understand their perspective.

  Example: Mark and Laura have a disagreement about finances. Mark takes a step back and tries to understand Laura's perspective, realizing that her concerns are valid and that they can work together to find a solution.

- **Using Humor to Diffuse Tension:** Use humor to lighten the mood and diffuse tension.

  Example: Emily and Jack are in the middle of a heated argument when Jack suddenly makes a funny comment, breaking the tension and allowing them to laugh and continue the conversation in a more positive tone.

- **Seeking Outside Help When Needed (Couples Therapy)** : Don't be afraid to seek outside help when communication barriers become too great to overcome on your own.

  Example: David and Rachel have been struggling to communicate effectively and decide to seek the help of a couples therapist. With the therapist's guidance, they learn new communication skills and strategies to improve their relationship.

- **Recognizing and Managing Stress and Anxiety:**Recognize how stress and anxiety can impact communication and take steps to manage them.

  Example: James and Leah notice that they tend to communicate more effectively when they're both relaxed and not stressed. They make a conscious effort to manage their stress and anxiety levels, prioritizing self-care and relaxation techniques.

- **Building Trust and Loyalty:** Work to build trust and loyalty in your relationship, which can help overcome communication barriers.

  Example: Samantha and Michael prioritize building trust and loyalty by being transparent and honest with each other, following through on commitments, and showing appreciation and gratitude.

- **Creating a Supportive and Non-Judgmental Space for Communication:** Create a safe and supportive environment where both partners feel comfortable communicating openly and honestly.

  Example: Emily and Jack create a "safe space" for communication by setting aside dedicated time to talk, free from distractions and judgment.

- **Enhances Emotional Intimacy :** Effective communication helps build emotional intimacy, creating a deeper connection and understanding between partners.

Example: Sarah and Mike have an open and honest conversation about their feelings and desires, leading to a stronger emotional bond and increased intimacy.

- **Promotes Conflict Resolution :** Effective communication helps resolve conflicts in a healthy and constructive manner, preventing resentment and strengthening the relationship.

Example: Emily and Jack have a disagreement, but they communicate effectively, listening to each other's perspectives and finding a resolution that works for both.

- **Supports Personal Growth and Development :** Effective communication encourages personal growth and development, helping individuals understand their needs and desires.

Example: David and his partner, Rachel, have open conversations about their goals and aspirations, supporting each other's personal growth and development.

- **Encourages Honesty and Transparency :** Effective communication promotes honesty and transparency, building trust and strengthening the relationship.

Example: Mark and Laura have a conversation about their financial concerns, being honest and transparent about their spending habits and working together to find a solution .

- **Fosters a Sense of Trust and Loyalty** : Effective communication builds trust and loyalty, creating a sense of security and stability in the relationship.

  Example: James and Leah have open and honest conversations, building trust and loyalty and strengthening their relationship.

- **Helps Navigate Life's Challenges and Transitions** : Effective communication helps navigate life's challenges and transitions, such as moving in together or starting a family.

  Example: Samantha and Michael have open conversations about their plans for the future, navigating the challenges of starting a family and building a strong foundation for their relationship.

- **Strengthens Bond and Connection** : Effective communication strengthens the bond and connection between partners, creating a more fulfilling and satisfying relationship.

  Example: Emily and Jack have regular date nights, communicating effectively and strengthening their bond and connection.

- **Encourages Active Listening and Understanding**:Effective communication encourages active listening and understanding, helping partners truly hear and understand each other's needs and desires.

  Example: David and Rachel practice active listening, making eye contact and clarifying their understanding of each other's needs and desires.

Chapter

2

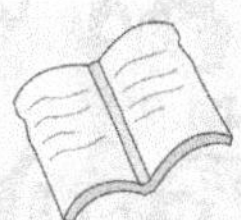

Chapter Outline

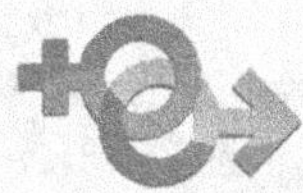

- Sexual desire
- Sexual frequency, initiation & preference
- Sexual positions, touch, Active listening
- Sexual health, wellness & hygiene
- Sexual disfunction & treatment

- Sexual desire and arousal
- Sexual intimacy, connection & feedback
- Sexual boundaries & consent
- Sex trauma and healing
- Sexual pleasure, fantasy & desire

As we delve into the intricacies of building a strong and healthy relationship, it is essential to acknowledge the significance of understanding your partner's sexual needs. Sexual education is a vital aspect of any romantic relationship, and grasping your partner's sexual desires, preferences, and boundaries is crucial for a fulfilling connection. In this chapter, we will explore the various facets of understanding your partner's sexual needs, including sexual desire, sexual preferences, and communication.

★ Sexual Desire

Sexual desire is a fundamental aspect of human sexuality, and understanding your partner's sexual desire is essential to meeting their sexual needs. Sexual desire can vary greatly from person to person, and it is crucial to recognize that your partner's desire may differ from yours. Understanding and respecting these differences can help create a more harmonious and satisfying sexual connection.

★ Sexual Frequency

One aspect of sexual desire is frequency. Your partner may have a different frequency of sexual desire than you, and understanding their needs and finding a mutually comfortable frequency is crucial. It is essential to communicate openly and honestly about your desires and boundaries, ensuring that both partners feel comfortable and satisfied.

Example: If your partner has a higher sexual desire than you, finding ways to compromise and meet their needs while also respecting your own boundaries is essential. This may involve exploring new ways to connect intimately, such as through touch or other forms of intimacy.

★ Sexual Initiation

Another aspect of sexual desire is initiation. Your partner may have different preferences for initiating sexual activity, and understanding their needs and boundaries is vital. It is essential to communicate openly and honestly about your desires and boundaries, ensuring that both partners feel comfortable and respected.

Example: If your partner prefers to initiate sexual activity, respecting their boundaries and communicating your own needs is essential. This may involve discussing your desires and boundaries openly and honestly, ensuring that both partners feel comfortable and respected.

★ Sexual Preferences

Sexual preferences play a significant role in understanding your partner's sexual needs. These preferences can include various aspects, such as sexual positions, touch, and intimacy. Understanding and respecting your partner's preferences can help create a more fulfilling and satisfying sexual connection.

★ Sex Positions

Your partner may have preferred sexual positions that provide comfort and pleasure. Understanding their needs and exploring new positions together can enhance your sexual connection. It is essential to communicate openly and honestly about your desires and boundaries, ensuring that both partners feel comfortable and respected.

Example: If your partner prefers a specific sexual position, exploring new ways to make that position comfortable and enjoyable for both of you can strengthen your sexual bond. This may involve experimenting with new positions or finding ways to modify existing positions to suit both partners' needs.

★ Touch

Your partner may have specific preferences for touch and intimacy. Understanding their needs and boundaries is essential, and communicating openly and honestly about your desires and boundaries can help create a more intimate and comfortable connection.

Example: If your partner prefers gentle touch, respecting their boundaries and communicating your own needs can create a more intimate and comfortable connection. This may involve discussing your desires and boundaries openly and honestly, ensuring that both partners feel comfortable and respected.

★ Sexual Communication

Communication is key in understanding your partner's sexual needs. Communicating openly and honestly about your desires, boundaries, and preferences can help create a more fulfilling and satisfying sexual connection.

★ Open Communication

Communicating openly and honestly about your sexual needs and desires is vital. It is essential to create a safe and supportive environment where both partners feel comfortable discussing their desires and boundaries.

Example: Having an open and honest conversation about your sexual needs and desires can help you better understand your partner's needs and create a more fulfilling sexual connection. This may involve discussing your desires, boundaries, and preferences openly and honestly, ensuring that both partners feel comfortable and respected.

★ Active Listening

Listening actively to your partner's needs and desires is essential. It is crucial to create a safe and supportive environment where both partners feel comfortable discussing their desires and boundaries.

Example: When your partner shares their sexual needs and desires, actively listening and responding with empathy and understanding can create a safe and supportive environment for sexual exploration. This may involve maintaining eye contact, asking clarifying questions, and responding with understanding and empathy.

★ Sexual Desire and Arousal

Understanding your partner's sexual desire and arousal is crucial in building a strong and healthy relationship. It's important to be aware of their needs and desires and to be supportive of their sexual health.

Example: If your partner has a low libido, be supportive and understanding of their needs. Encourage them to seek professional help and be patient with their healing process.

★ Sexual Intimacy and Connection

Sexual intimacy and connection are crucial in building a strong and healthy relationship. It's important to be aware of your partner's needs and desires and to be supportive of their sexual health.

Example: If your partner desires more intimacy and connection, be supportive and understanding of their needs. Encourage them to express their desires and boundaries and be patient with their healing process.

★ Sexual Communication and Feedback

Sexual communication and feedback are crucial in building a strong and healthy relationship. It's important to be aware of your partner's needs and desires and to be supportive of their sexual health.

Example: If your partner desires more communication and feedback during sexual activity, be supportive and understanding of their needs. Encourage them to express their desires and boundaries and be patient with their healing process.

★ Sexual Exploration and Experimentation

Sexual exploration and experimentation can be a fun and exciting way to build a strong and healthy relationship. It's important to be aware of your partner's needs and desires and to be supportive of their sexual health.

Example: If your partner desires to explore new sexual experiences, be supportive and understanding of their needs. Encourage them to express their desires and boundaries and be patient with their healing process.

★ Sexual Boundaries and Consent

Sexual boundaries and consent are crucial in building a strong and healthy relationship. It's important to be aware of your partner's needs and desires and to be supportive of their sexual health.

Example: If your partner has boundaries around sexual activity, be supportive and understanding of their needs. Encourage them to express their desires and boundaries and be patient with their healing process.

★ Sexual Health and Wellness

Sexual health and wellness are crucial in building a strong and healthy relationship. It's important to be aware of your partner's needs and desires and to be supportive of their sexual health.

Example: If your partner has concerns around sexual health and wellness, be supportive and understanding of their needs. Encourage them to seek professional help and be patient with their healing process.

★ Sexual Trauma and Healing

Sexual trauma can have a profound impact on a person's sexual health and well-being. Understanding your partner's experiences and being supportive of their healing process is crucial in building a strong and healthy relationship.

Example: If your partner has experienced sexual trauma, be supportive and understanding of their needs. Encourage them to seek professional help and be patient with their healing process.

★ Sexual Orientation and Gender Identity

Understanding your partner's sexual orientation and gender identity is crucial in building a strong and healthy relationship. It's important to be respectful and supportive of their identity and to create a safe and welcoming environment for them to express themselves.

Example: If your partner identifies as LGBTQ+, be supportive and respectful of their identity. Use their preferred pronouns and create a safe space for them to express themselves.

★ Sexual Pleasure and Satisfaction

Sexual pleasure and satisfaction are crucial in building a strong and healthy relationship. It's important to be aware of your partner's needs and desires and to be supportive of their sexual health.

Example: If your partner desires more pleasure and satisfaction during sexual activity, be supportive and understanding of their needs. Encourage them to express their desires and boundaries and be patient with their healing process.

★ Sexual Conflict and Resolution

Sexual conflict and resolution are crucial in building a strong and healthy relationship. It's important to be aware of your partner's needs and desires and to be supportive of their sexual health.

Example: If you and your partner experience sexual conflict, be supportive and understanding of their needs. Encourage open and honest communication and work together to find a resolution that works for both of you.

★ Sexual Fantasies and Desires

Understanding your partner's sexual fantasies and desires can help you better understand their needs and preferences.

Example: If your partner shares their sexual fantasies with you, listen with an open mind and be supportive of their desires.

★ Sexual Positions and Techniques

Understanding different sexual positions and techniques can help you better please your partner and improve your overall sexual experience.

Example: If your partner enjoys a specific sexual position, be willing to try it and ask for feedback on how to improve.

★ Sexual Communication During Intimacy

Communication during intimacy is crucial in building a strong and healthy relationship. It's important to be aware of your partner's needs and desires and to communicate openly and honestly.

Example: If you and your partner are intimate, communicate openly and honestly about your desires and boundaries.

★ Sexual Intimacy and Emotional Connection

Sexual intimacy and emotional connection are crucial in building a strong and healthy relationship. It's important to be aware of your partner's needs and desires and to prioritize emotional connection.

Example: If your partner desires more emotional connection during intimacy, be supportive and understanding of their needs.

★ Sexual Health and Hygiene

Sexual health and hygiene are crucial in building a strong and healthy relationship. It's important to be aware of your partner's needs and desires and to prioritize sexual health.

Example: If your partner has concerns around sexual health and hygiene, be supportive and understanding of their needs.

★ Sexual Dysfunction and Treatment

Sexual dysfunction can affect anyone, and it's important to be understanding and supportive of your partner's needs.

Example: If your partner experiences sexual dysfunction, be supportive and understanding of their needs. Encourage them to seek professional help and be patient with their healing process.

★ Sexual Pleasure and Pain

Sexual pleasure and pain can be a complex topic, and it's important to be aware of your partner's needs and desires.

Example: If your partner experiences pain during sexual activity, be supportive and understanding of their needs. Encourage them to seek professional help and be patient with their healing process.

Chapter
3

 **Chapter Outline** 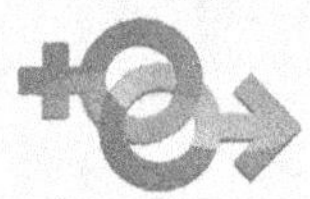

- Foundation of sexual intimacy
- Emotional connect for intimacy
- Exploration flame of intimacy
- Foreplay prelude & passion
- Mutual satisfaction pillar of intimacy
- Respect and consent
- Post intimacy connection
- Enhancing sexual wellbeing

Intimacy is an essential aspect of any romantic relationship, and sexual satisfaction plays a significant role in this domain. Understanding and fulfilling your partner's sexual needs can strengthen your bond, foster deeper emotional connections, and enhance the overall quality of your relationship. This chapter delves into the various elements that contribute to a satisfying sexual relationship, providing insights and practical tips to help you and your partner achieve a fulfilling intimate life.

★ **Communication: The Foundation of Sexual Intimacy**

- **Effective Communication :** Open and honest communication is the cornerstone of a healthy sexual relationship. Discussing your desires, boundaries, and fantasies can lead to a more satisfying sexual experience. Here's how to approach it:

- **Create a Safe Space :** Ensure that your conversations about sex occur in a judgment-free zone. Encourage openness and vulnerability.

- **Use "I" Statements :** Frame your desires and concerns using "I" statements to express how you feel without blaming your partner. For example, "I feel more connected when we spend time on foreplay."

- **Active Listening :** Pay attention to your partner's words and respond thoughtfully. Show empathy and understanding.

- **Regular Check-Ins :** Regularly checking in with each other about your sexual relationship can prevent misunderstandings and keep the lines of communication open. Set aside time to discuss what's working, what's not, and any new desires or concerns.

★ **Emotional Connection: The Heart of Intimacy**

- **Building Trust :** A strong emotional bond is the bedrock of sexual intimacy. Trust is built through consistent, loving actions and clear communication. Here are some ways to strengthen your emotional connection:

- **Quality Time :** Spend time together doing activities you both enjoy. This can range from simple daily routines to special dates.

- **Meaningful Conversations :** Engage in deep and meaningful conversations. Share your dreams, fears, and life goals.

- **Affection :** Show physical and verbal affection regularly. Small gestures like holding hands, hugging, and saying "I love you" can significantly enhance your bond.

- **Emotional Vulnerability :** Allowing yourself to be vulnerable with your partner fosters intimacy. Share your feelings and experiences honestly, and encourage your partner to do the same.

- The Importance of Foreplay : Foreplay is crucial for building arousal and anticipation. It helps both partners feel more connected and engaged. Here's how to make the most of foreplay:

- **Take Your Time :** Don't rush. Spend ample time on kissing, touching, and exploring each other's bodies.

- **Sensual Touch :** Use gentle, sensual touches to stimulate erogenous zones. Vary the pressure and pace to keep things exciting.

- **Verbal Arousal:** Whisper sweet nothings or express your desires verbally. Hearing your partner's voice can be incredibly arousing.

- **Experimentation in Foreplay :** Experiment with different types of foreplay to find what excites you both. This could include massage, oral sex, or using erotic toys.

★ Exploration: Keeping the Flame Alive

- **Variety and Experimentation :** Variety is key to maintaining excitement in your sexual relationship. Be open to trying new things together:

- **New Positions :** Experiment with different sexual positions to find what feels best for both of you.

- **Erotic Toys :** Introduce toys to add a new dimension to your sexual experience. Discuss and choose toys that interest both of you.

- **Role-Playing :** Role-playing can add a fun and imaginative element to your intimacy. Discuss and set boundaries beforehand.

- **Mutual Exploration** : Exploration should be a mutual journey. Ensure that both partners are comfortable and willing to try new things. Respect each other's boundaries and preferences.

★ Focus on Pleasure: Mutual Satisfaction

- **Prioritizing Pleasure** : Focus on the pleasure and satisfaction of both partners rather than solely on the act itself. Here's how:

    - **Attentive Listening** : Pay attention to your partner's physical and verbal cues. Adjust your actions based on their responses.

    - **Feedback** : Encourage your partner to provide feedback. This can be done during or after the experience to enhance future encounters.

    - **Balance** : Balance giving and receiving pleasure Ensure that both partners have their needs met.

    - **Mindfulness and Presence** : Being fully present during intimate moments enhances the experience. Practice mindfulness by focusing on the sensations, emotions, and connection with your partner.

★ Respect and Consent: The Pillars of Safe Intimacy

- **Establishing Consent** : Consent is non-negotiable in any sexual relationship. Here's how to ensure a consensual experience:

    - **Clear Communication** : Discuss and agree on boundaries and limits beforehand.

- **Ongoing Consent** : Consent should be ongoing. Check in with your partner regularly to ensure they are comfortable and willing to continue.

- **Respecting Boundaries** : Always respect your partner's boundaries. If they express discomfort, stop immediately and discuss how to proceed.

- **Creating a Safe Environment** : A safe and respectful environment is crucial for intimacy. Ensure that both partners feel valued and respected at all times.

★ **Aftercare: The Post-Intimacy Connection**

- **The Importance of Aftercare** : Aftercare is the period following sexual activity where partners connect and care for each other. It helps in solidifying the bond and ensuring emotional well-being. Here's what to consider:

- **Physical Comfort** : Cuddle, hold hands, or simply lie close to each other. Physical closeness reinforces emotional connection.

- **Verbal Reassurance** : Express love and appreciation. Compliment your partner and share positive feelings about the experience.

- **Emotional Support** : Be attentive to your partner's emotional state. Offer comfort and support if needed.

- **Tailoring Aftercare** : Aftercare can vary from couple to couple. Discuss and understand each other's needs to tailor the aftercare experience accordingly.

★ **Physical Health: Enhancing Sexual Well-Being**

- **Maintaining Good Health :** Good physical health directly impacts sexual performance and satisfaction. Consider the following aspects:

- **Regular Exercise :** Exercise improves stamina, flexibility, and overall energy levels.

- **Balanced Diet :** A nutritious diet supports overall health and vitality. Include foods that boost libido and energy.

- **Adequate Rest :** Ensure you get enough sleep to maintain energy levels and mood.

- **Addressing Health Issues :** If you experience any health issues that affect your sexual relationship, seek professional advice. Addressing physical or psychological concerns can significantly improve your intimate life.

Conclusion

Intimacy is a multifaceted journey that requires effort, understanding, and mutual respect. By focusing on communication, emotional connection, foreplay, exploration, pleasure, respect, consent, aftercare, and physical health, you can create a deeply satisfying and fulfilling sexual relationship. Remember, intimacy is an ongoing process of learning and growing together, so be patient and enjoy the journey with your partner.

Exploring Sexual Pleasure & Desire

Chapter Outline

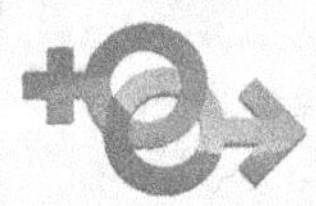

- Nature of sexual pleasure
- Types of sexual pleasure
- Nature of sexual desire
- Types of sexual desire
- Safe sex practices
- Communicating About Sex

Exploring sexual pleasure and desire are essential components of human sexuality, profoundly influencing relationships, self-esteem, and overall well-being. This chapter explores the intricate dimensions of sexual pleasure and desire, examining their biological, psychological, cultural, and social underpinnings. Understanding these aspects can enhance intimacy, foster healthy sexual relationships, and promote a positive sense of sexual self.

★ The Nature of Sexual Pleasure

Sexual pleasure is a positive emotional and physical response to sexual stimuli. It involves sensory experiences, emotional connection, and psychological fulfillment. The sensation of sexual pleasure varies among individuals and can be influenced by numerous factors.

1.   Biological Basis

Sexual pleasure is rooted in the nervous system, where sensory receptors send signals to the brain, resulting in pleasurable sensations. Key biological components include:

- **Neurotransmitters and Hormones :** Dopamine, serotonin, and oxytocin play significant roles in the experience of sexual pleasure. Dopamine is associated with the reward system, serotonin contributes to mood regulation, and oxytocin fosters bonding and intimacy.

- **Genital Stimulation :** Physical stimulation of erogenous zones, such as the genitals, breasts, and other sensitive areas, triggers the release of these chemicals, enhancing sexual pleasure.

2.   Psychological Factors

Psychological factors significantly influence sexual pleasure. These include:

- **Emotional Connection : A** strong emotional bond with a partner can enhance the intensity of sexual pleasure.

- **Mental State :** Stress, anxiety, and self-esteem can affect the ability to experience sexual pleasure. A relaxed and positive mental state is conducive to pleasurable experiences.

- **Sexual Fantasies and Desires :** Personal fantasies and desires can amplify sexual arousal and pleasure.

★ Types of Sexual Pleasure

Sexual pleasure can manifest in various forms:

- **Physical Pleasure** : Derived from the tactile sensations of touch, caressing, and sexual intercourse.

- **Emotional Pleasure** : Arising from feelings of love, intimacy, and connection with a partner.

- **Intellectual Pleasure** : Stimulated by erotic conversations, fantasies, and mental engagement.

★ The Nature of Sexual Desire

Sexual desire is a motivational state that drives individuals to seek sexual activity and experiences. It can be spontaneous or responsive and is influenced by a complex interplay of biological, psychological, and social factors.

Biological Underpinnings

The biological basis of sexual desire involves:

- **Hormones** : Testosterone and estrogen are crucial in regulating sexual desire. Testosterone, present in both men and women, plays a significant role in libido. Estrogen influences desire, particularly in women, through its effects on mood and vaginal lubrication.

- **Brain Activity** : Areas such as the hypothalamus and limbic system are involved in the regulation of sexual desire. These brain regions process sensory information and emotional responses, driving the urge for sexual activity.

Psychological Influences

Psychological factors affecting sexual desire include:

- **Personality and Temperament :** Individual differences in personality can influence levels of sexual desire. For instance, people who are more open to new experiences may have higher levels of sexual curiosity.

- **Mental Health :** Conditions such as depression, anxiety, and past trauma can impact sexual desire. Addressing mental health issues can help in restoring a healthy level of desire.

- **Relationship Dynamics :** The quality of a relationship, including communication, trust, and emotional closeness, significantly affects sexual desire.

★ **Types of Sexual Desire**

Sexual desire can be classified into:

- **Spontaneous Desire :** Arises suddenly and without any apparent external stimulus.

- **Responsive Desire :** Emerges in response to sexual stimuli or context, such as physical touch or a romantic setting.

★ **The Interplay Between Sexual Pleasure and Desire**

Sexual pleasure and desire are interconnected in a dynamic relationship, where the fulfillment of desire leads to pleasure, and pleasurable experiences can enhance future desires.

- **Positive Feedback Loop**

Engaging in pleasurable sexual activities can create a positive feedback loop, where the enjoyment of the experience reinforces the desire for similar activities in the future.

- **Anticipation and Arousal**

Anticipation of sexual activity can heighten arousal and intensify the subsequent pleasure. The brain's reward system is activated not only by the act itself but also by the expectation, increasing overall satisfaction.

- **Challenges and Discrepancies**

Discrepancies in sexual desire between partners can pose challenges. Open communication, understanding each other's needs, and seeking professional help when necessary can address these issues and promote a harmonious sexual relationship.

- **Cultural and Social Influences**

Cultural and social contexts profoundly shape perceptions and expressions of sexual pleasure and desire. Norms, values, and societal attitudes play crucial roles in defining acceptable sexual behaviors.

- **Cultural Norms and Values**

Different cultures have diverse norms regarding sexuality. These norms influence:

  - **Expression of Desire** : Some cultures may encourage open expression of sexual desires, while others may impose restrictions.

- **Sexual Education** : Access to comprehensive sexual education varies, affecting knowledge and attitudes towards sexual pleasure and health.

- **Media and Popular Culture**

Media and popular culture can both positively and negatively influence sexual attitudes:

- **Positive Influence** : Representation of diverse sexual experiences and orientations can promote inclusivity and acceptance.

- **Negative Influence** : Unrealistic portrayals of sex can create harmful stereotypes and expectations, leading to dissatisfaction and pressure.

- **Social Constructs and Gender Roles**

Gender roles and social constructs significantly impact sexual desire and pleasure:

- **Expectations and Norms** : Traditional gender roles often dictate acceptable sexual behaviors and desires, potentially limiting individual expression.

- **Power Dynamics** : Power imbalances in relationships can affect the ability to experience and communicate sexual needs.

★ **The Pursuit of Sexual Pleasure and Desire**

The pursuit of sexual pleasure and desire is a natural and healthy aspect of human life. However, it is essential to approach this pursuit with mindfulness and respect for oneself and others.

- **Communication and Consent**

Effective communication and mutual consent are foundational to a healthy sexual relationship. Discussing desires, boundaries, and preferences openly can enhance intimacy and ensure that both partners feel respected and fulfilled.

- **Exploring Sexuality**

Exploring one's sexuality can lead to greater self-awareness and satisfaction. This exploration can include:

- **Self-Exploration :** Understanding one's own body, desires, and boundaries through masturbation and self-reflection.

- **Shared Exploration :** Engaging in activities with a partner to discover mutual pleasures and deepen emotional connection.

- **Addressing Sexual Issues**

Sexual issues such as low desire, performance anxiety, or dissatisfaction are common. Addressing these issues through open communication, counseling, or therapy can improve sexual well-being and relationship satisfaction.

- **Ethical and Safe Practices**

The pursuit of sexual pleasure and desire should be guided by ethical considerations and a commitment to safety.

- **Respect and Boundaries**

Respecting personal and partner boundaries is crucial. Understanding and honoring consent is fundamental to any sexual interaction .

- **Safe Sex Practices**

Practicing safe sex is essential to prevent sexually transmitted infections (STIs) and unwanted pregnancies. This includes using condoms, regular STI testing, and open discussions about sexual health with partners.

- **Emotional Well-being**

Balancing physical pleasure with emotional well-being ensures a holistic approach to sexuality. Prioritizing emotional health, addressing mental health issues, and seeking support when needed contribute to a satisfying sexual life.

Conclusion

Exploring sexual pleasure and desire reveals their profound impact on human relationships and individual well-being. By understanding the biological, psychological, cultural, and social dimensions, individuals can navigate their sexual lives with confidence and respect. Embracing open communication, mutual consent, and ethical practices can lead to fulfilling and meaningful sexual experiences, enhancing overall quality of life.

Chapter

5

Chapter Outline

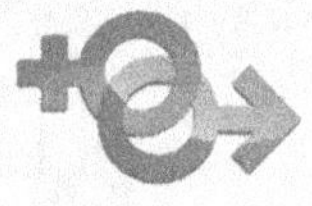

- ❑ Importance of communication
- ❑ Benifit of sex positions
- ❑ Ethical considerations & Mutual respect
- ❑ Respecting individual differences

- ❑ Basic sex positions
- ❑ Advance sex positions
- ❑ Sex Position customisation
- ❑ Consent and mutual agreement

Sexual satisfaction is a crucial aspect of a healthy relationship. Exploring different sex positions can enhance intimacy, pleasure, and connection between partners. This chapter focuses on various sex positions designed to satisfy your partner, considering their physical, emotional, and psychological aspects. Effective communication, consent, and mutual respect are essential in achieving sexual satisfaction.

★ **The Importance of Communication**

Open and honest dialogue about sexual preferences, boundaries, and desires ensures that both partners feel comfortable and respected. Before experimenting with different sex positions, discuss what each partner enjoys and dislikes in bed, establish boundaries, and maintain ongoing communication to adapt to changing preferences.

★ Basic Sex Positions and Their Benefits

Understanding basic sex positions provides a foundation for exploring more advanced variations. These positions cater to different levels of intimacy, control, and stimulation.

Missionary Position

The missionary position is a classic where one partner lies on their back while the other lies on top.

- **Benefits** : Allows for deep penetration, face-to-face intimacy, and easy adjustment for clitoral stimulation.

- **Tips** : Adjust the angle of penetration by placing a pillow under the hips for increased comfort and pleasure.

Woman on Top (Cowgirl)

In this position, the woman straddles her partner, controlling the angle and depth of penetration.

- **Benefits** : Empowers the receiving partner to control the pace and depth, facilitating clitoral stimulation and emotional connection.

- **Variations** : The woman can face forward (cowgirl) or backward (reverse cowgirl) for different sensations.

Doggy Style

Doggy style involves one partner kneeling on all fours while the other partner penetrates from behind.

- Benefits : Allows for deep penetration and easy access to the G-spot. It also provides a visually stimulating angle.

- Tips : Communication about the angle and speed can prevent discomfort and enhance pleasure.

Spooning

In the spooning position, both partners lie on their sides, facing the same direction, with the penetrating partner behind.

- **Benefits** : Offers a gentle, intimate experience with full-body contact. Ideal for slow, sensual lovemaking.

- **Tips.** : Adjust the angle by bending or straightening the legs to find the most comfortable and pleasurable position.

★ **Advanced Sex Positions for Enhanced Pleasure**

Exploring more advanced positions can add variety and excitement to a sexual relationship. These positions often require greater flexibility and strength but can offer unique sensations and deeper intimacy.

The Lotus

In the lotus position, one partner sits cross-legged while the other straddles their lap, wrapping their legs around the seated partner.

- Benefits : Promotes deep emotional connection through face-to-face contact and synchronized movement. Allows for deep penetration and intimate clitoral stimulation.

- Tips : Support each other to maintain balance and take breaks as needed.

Standing Positions

Standing positions involve both partners standing, with one partner lifting the other or leaning against a wall for support.

- Benefits : Provides opportunities for spontaneous and adventurous sex. Allows for deep penetration and unique angles.
- Tips : Use furniture or walls for support to maintain stability and comfort.

The Bridge

In the bridge position, one partner lies on their back, lifting their hips off the ground to form a bridge while the other partner penetrates from above.

- **Benefits** : Offers deep penetration and G-spot stimulation. The elevated hips can enhance sensations for both partners.

- **Tips** : Ensure comfort by supporting the back and hips with pillows or taking breaks to avoid strain.

The Butterfly

In the butterfly position, the receiving partner lies on their back with their legs raised and resting on their partner's shoulders while the penetrating partner stands or kneels at the edge of the bed.

- **Benefits** : Allows for deep penetration and easy clitoral stimulation. Provides a visually appealing angle for the penetrating partner.

- **Tips** : Adjust the height of the bed or use pillows to enhance comfort and accessibility.

Customizing Positions for Maximum Satisfaction

Customizing sex positions to suit personal preferences and physical abilities can enhance satisfaction. Incorporate pillows, wedges, and other props to provide support and enhance angles, and adapt positions to accommodate physical limitations or disabilities.

Ethical Considerations and Mutual Respect

Ethical considerations and mutual respect are paramount in any sexual relationship. Ensuring that both partners feel valued and respected is crucial for a healthy and fulfilling sex life.

Consent and Mutual Agreement

Consent is the cornerstone of any sexual activity. Both partners should enthusiastically agree to engage in sexual activities and feel free to express their boundaries at any time.

Respecting Individual Differences

Each person has unique preferences, desires, and boundaries. Respecting these differences and being open to compromise fosters a positive sexual relationship.

Conclusion

Exploring different sex positions   significantly enhance sexual satisfaction and intimacy between partners. By emphasizing communication, customization, and mutual respect, couples can discover what works best for them and create a fulfilling sexual relationship. Remember, the key to satisfying your partner lies in understanding their needs, being open to experimentation, and fostering a deep emotional connection.

 **Chapter Outline** 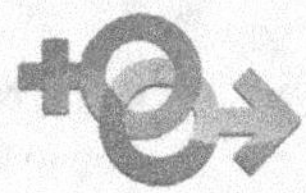

- ❏ Understanding foreplay
- ❏ Importance of communication during foreplay
- ❏ Foreplay tricks and techniques
- ❏ Steps of foreplay

Foreplay is a crucial aspect of intimacy and sexual satisfaction, setting the stage for a more connected and pleasurable experience. It's about building anticipation, increasing arousal, and deepening the emotional bond between partners. This chapter explores various steps and techniques of foreplay to enhance intimacy and satisfaction.

★ Understanding Foreplay

Foreplay isn't just a precursor to sex; it's an essential part of the sexual experience itself. It involves a range of physical and emotional activities that stimulate and arouse both partners. The goal is to build a strong connection and ensure that both partners feel loved, valued, and ready for further intimacy.

★ The Importance of Communication

Open and honest communication is the foundation of satisfying foreplay. Discussing likes, dislikes, boundaries, and desires helps partners understand each other's needs and preferences. Here are some tips for effective communication:

- **Express Your Desires :** hare what you enjoy and what turns you on.

- **Ask for Feedback :** Encourage your partner to communicate their feelings and preferences.

- **Be Respectful :** Respect each other's boundaries and comfort levels.

- **Listen Actively :** Pay attention to verbal and non-verbal cues to gauge your partner's enjoyment.

★ Steps and Techniques for Foreplay

1. Setting the Mood

Creating the right atmosphere can significantly enhance the foreplay experience. Here are some ideas to set the mood:

- **Lighting :** Dim the lights or use candles to create a romantic ambiance.

- **Music :** Play soft, sensual music to relax and arouse.

- **Aromatherapy :** Use scented candles or essential oils to stimulate the senses.

- **Comfort :** Ensure the environment is comfortable and free from distractions.

2. Start with Gentle Touch

Physical touch is a powerful way to build arousal and intimacy. Begin with gentle, non-sexual touches to gradually increase excitement:

- **Holding Hands :** A simple yet intimate gesture that fosters connection.

- **Caressing :** Softly stroke your partner's arms, back, or face.

- **Hugging :** A warm embrace can create a sense of security and closeness.

- **Kissing :** Start with gentle kisses on the lips, cheeks, or neck.

3. Focus on Sensual Kissing

Kissing is an essential part of foreplay that can significantly enhance arousal:

- **Soft Kisses:** Begin with light, tender kisses on the lips.

- **Deep Kisses :** Gradually progress to deeper, more passionate kisses.

- **Exploration :** Kiss other sensitive areas like the neck, earlobes, and collarbone.

- **Variety :** Mix up the intensity and pace to keep things exciting.

4. Use Your Hands

Hands can be incredibly effective in stimulating your partner:

- **Massage :** Give your partner a sensual massage to relax and arouse them. Focus on areas like the back, shoulders, and legs.

- **Caressing :** Gently caress your partner's body, paying attention to erogenous zones.

- **Light Touches :** Use light, feathery touches to create anticipation and excitement.

5. Oral Stimulation

Oral stimulation can be intensely pleasurable and is a key component of foreplay:

- **Lips and Tongue :** Use your lips and tongue to kiss, lick, and tease your partner's body.

- **Erogenous Zones :** Pay attention to sensitive areas like the neck, nipples, inner thighs, and genitals.

- **Feedback :** Listen to your partner's responses and adjust your technique accordingly.

6. Explore Erogenous Zones

Erogenous zones are areas of the body that are particularly sensitive to touch and can enhance arousal:

- **Neck and Ears :** Gently kiss and nibble on your partner's neck and ears.

- **Breasts and Nipples :** Caress, kiss, and gently suckle the breasts and nipples.

- Inner Thighs : Use light touches and kisses on the inner thighs to build anticipation.

- Lower Back and Buttocks : Caress and massage these areas to increase arousal.

7. Engage in Sensual Play

Incorporate playful activities to add variety and excitement to foreplay:

- **Role-Playing :** Experiment with different roles and scenarios to explore fantasies.

- **Teasing :** Lightly tease your partner by touching and then pulling away to build anticipation.

- **Eye Contact :** Maintain eye contact to deepen the emotional connection and enhance arousal.

8. Use Toys and Props

Introducing toys and props can add a new dimension to foreplay:

- **Vibrators :** Use vibrators to stimulate erogenous zones and enhance pleasure.

- **Blindfolds :** Blindfolds can heighten the senses and create a sense of mystery.

- **Feathers and Silk Scarves :** Use feathers and silk scarves for light, teasing touches.

9. Take Your Time

Foreplay should not be rushed. Taking your time allows both partners to fully enjoy and savor the experience:

- **Patience :** Be patient and focus on the journey rather than the destination.

- **Slow Down :** Slow, deliberate movements can heighten anticipation and arousal.

- **Enjoy the Moment :** Focus on the sensations and the emotional connection with your partner.

10. Emotional Intimacy

Emotional intimacy is just as important as physical stimulation in foreplay:

- **Affection :** Show affection through words and actions.

- **Compliments :** Compliment your partner and make them feel valued and desired.

- **Connection :** Share intimate thoughts and feelings to deepen your bond.

Conclusion

Foreplay is an essential part of a satisfying sexual experience. By focusing on communication, setting the right mood, and exploring various techniques, you can enhance intimacy and pleasure for both you and your partner. Remember that foreplay is about mutual enjoyment and connection, so take the time to understand and fulfill each other's desires.

Sex Pleasuring Devices & Materials

 **Chapter Outline** 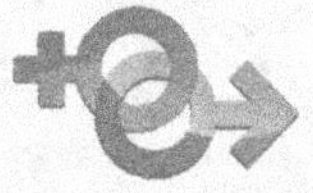

- Understanding sex pleasuring devices
- Vibrator dilbos anal toys

- Material for sex pleasuring devices
- Enhancing the experience using sex devices

Sexual intimacy is a crucial aspect of human relationships, providing both physical pleasure and emotional connection. In the modern world, sex pleasuring devices and materials are widely available and can enhance the sexual experiences of individuals and couples. This chapter explores the various types of sex toys and materials designed to satisfy your partner, offering insights into their benefits, proper use, and considerations for ensuring a safe and enjoyable experience.

★ Understanding Sex Pleasuring Devices

Sex pleasuring devices, commonly referred to as sex toys, are objects or tools used to enhance sexual pleasure. These devices can be used alone or with a partner to stimulate erogenous zones, increase arousal, and facilitate orgasm. They come in various shapes, sizes, and functionalities to cater to different preferences and needs.

★ Vibrators

Vibrators are one of the most popular sex toys, known for their ability to provide intense stimulation through vibration. They come in different forms, such as bullet vibrators, wand vibrators, and rabbit vibrators. Vibrators can be used for clitoral, vaginal, or anal stimulation, making them versatile tools for sexual pleasure.

Benefits:

- Enhance sexual pleasure and orgasm
- Useful for individuals with difficulty achieving orgasm
- Can be used during solo play or with a partner

Usage Tips:

- Start with a low setting and gradually increase intensity
- Use water-based lubricant to enhance comfort
- Communicate with your partner to ensure mutual enjoyment

★ Dildos

Dildos are non-vibrating sex toys designed to resemble the shape of a penis. They can be made from various materials, including silicone, glass, and metal. Dildos can be used for vaginal or anal penetration and are available in a range of sizes and shapes.

Benefits:

- Provide a realistic experience of penetration
- Can be used for G-spot or P-spot stimulation
- Available in a variety of textures and designs

Usage Tips:

Use plenty of lubricant to avoid discomfort

- Choose a size that matches your comfort level
- Clean thoroughly before and after use

★ **Anal Toys**

Anal toys are specifically designed for anal stimulation. These include butt plugs, anal beads, and prostate massagers. They are often tapered for easy insertion and can provide unique sensations due to the sensitivity of the anal region.

Benefits:

- Enhance pleasure during anal play
- Can stimulate the prostate gland (P-spot) in men
- Increase overall sexual arousal

Usage Tips:

- Use a generous amount of anal lubricant
- Start with smaller sizes and gradually increase
- Relax and communicate with your partner to avoid discomfort

★ **Materials for Sex Pleasuring Devices**

The materials used in sex toys can significantly affect the experience and safety. It is essential to choose body-safe materials that are non-toxic and easy to clean.

1. **Silicone**

Silicone is a popular material for sex toys due to its non-porous nature, making it easy to clean and sanitize. It is also hypoallergenic and provides a realistic feel.

Benefits:

- Safe for the body and easy to clean
- Durable and long-lasting
- Feels smooth and realistic

Care Tips:

- Clean with warm water and mild soap or a specialized toy cleaner
- Store in a cool, dry place away from other silicone toys

2. Glass

Glass toys are made from borosilicate glass, which is durable and body-safe. They are often used for temperature play, as they can be heated or cooled for added sensation.

Benefits:

- Non-porous and easy to clean
- Can be heated or cooled for temperature play
- Aesthetic appeal with various designs

Care Tips:

- Clean with warm water and mild soap
- Handle with care to avoid breakage
- Avoid extreme temperature changes to prevent cracking

3. Stainless Steel

Stainless steel toys are known for their weight and smooth texture. They are non-porous, hypoallergenic, and can also be used for temperature play.

Benefits:

- Durable and body-safe
- Can be heated or cooled for added sensation
- Provide a different tactile experience due to their weight

Care Tips:

- Clean with warm water and mild soap
- Avoid using with abrasive cleaners
- Store in a dry place to prevent tarnishing

★ **Enhancing the Experience**

Using sex toys can significantly enhance sexual pleasure, but it is essential to consider the overall experience, including communication, comfort, and consent.

1. Communication

Open communication with your partner is vital when introducing sex toys into your relationship. Discuss your desires, boundaries, and any concerns to ensure a positive and enjoyable experience for both partners.

Benefits:

- Builds trust and intimacy
- Ensures mutual consent and comfort
- Enhances overall sexual satisfaction

Tips:

- Discuss preferences and boundaries beforehand
- Check in with each other during use
- Be open to feedback and adjustments

2. Comfort and Safety

Ensuring comfort and safety is crucial when using sex toys. Choose toys that are appropriate for your experience level and always use plenty of lubricant to prevent discomfort or injury.

Benefits:

- Prevents discomfort and injury
- Enhances overall pleasure and satisfaction
- Ensures a safe and enjoyable experience

Tips:

- Start with smaller toys if you are a beginner
- Use water-based lubricant with silicone toys
- Clean toys thoroughly before and after use

3. Exploring Together

Exploring sex toys together can be an exciting and bonding experience for couples. Experiment with different toys, techniques, and settings to discover what brings the most pleasure to you and your partner.

Benefits:

- Deepens emotional and physical connection
- Encourages mutual exploration and discovery
- Increases overall sexual satisfaction

Tips:

- Take turns using toys on each other
- Try different types of toys and settings
- Communicate openly about what feels good

Conclusion

Sex pleasuring devices and materials offer a wide range of options to enhance sexual pleasure and satisfaction. By understanding the different types of toys, their benefits, and how to use them safely, you can create a more fulfilling and enjoyable sexual experience for you and your partner. Open communication, consent, and a willingness to explore together are key to maximizing the benefits of these devices and materials.

Condoms Pleasure & Safety

Chapter Outline

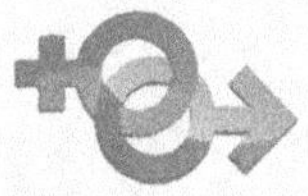

- ❑ Understanding Condoms
- ❑ History of condoms
- ❑ Types of condoms

- ❑ How to use condoms correctly
- ❑ Enhancing pleasure with condoms
- ❑ Addressing common concern

Condoms are one of the most widely used methods of contraception and protection against sexually transmitted infections (STIs). This chapter explores the various types of condoms, their correct usage, and how they can enhance sexual pleasure. Understanding these aspects can help individuals and couples make informed decisions about their sexual health and enjoyment.

★ Understanding Condoms

Condoms are barrier devices typically made from latex, polyurethane, or other materials. They are designed to cover the penis during sexual intercourse, preventing semen from entering the partner's body. This helps to reduce the risk of pregnancy and the transmission of STIs.

★ History of Condoms

The use of condoms dates back centuries, with evidence of their use in ancient civilizations. Early condoms were made from animal intestines or linen, but modern condoms are primarily made from latex or synthetic materials, offering greater reliability and comfort.

★ Types of Condoms

There are various types of condoms available, each catering to different needs and preferences. Understanding these types can help you choose the right condom for your sexual experience.

1. Latex Condoms

Latex condoms are the most common type, known for their elasticity, strength, and effectiveness in preventing pregnancy and STIs. They are widely available and come in various sizes, textures, and flavors.

Benefits:

- Highly effective at preventing pregnancy and STIs
- Widely available and affordable
- Elastic and durable

Considerations:

- Some individuals may have latex allergies
- Should be used with water-based or silicone-based lubricants (oil-based lubricants can degrade latex)

2. Polyurethane Condoms

Polyurethane condoms are made from a type of plastic and are an alternative for those with latex allergies. They are thinner than latex condoms, which can enhance sensitivity.

Benefits:

- Suitable for individuals with latex allergies
- Thinner, enhancing sensitivity
- Compatible with all types of lubricants

Considerations:

- Slightly less elastic than latex condoms
- May be more expensive than latex condoms

3. Polyisoprene Condoms

Polyisoprene condoms are another latex-free option, made from synthetic rubber. They offer similar benefits to latex condoms but without the risk of allergic reactions.

Benefits:

- Suitable for individuals with latex allergies
- Soft and flexible, providing a natural feel
- Effective in preventing pregnancy and STIs

Considerations:

- Slightly more expensive than latex condoms
- Should be used with water-based or silicone-based lubricants

4. Lambskin Condoms

Lambskin condoms are made from the intestinal membrane of lambs. They are effective at preventing pregnancy but do not protect against STIs due to their porous nature.

Benefits:

- Provides a natural feel
- Effective for contraception

Considerations:

- Does not protect against STIs
- More expensive and less widely available
- Not suitable for individuals with ethical or dietary concerns about animal products

5. Textured Condoms

Textured condoms, such as ribbed or dotted varieties, are designed to enhance pleasure by providing additional stimulation during intercourse.

Benefits:

- Enhances pleasure for both partners
- Available in various textures and patterns

Considerations:

- Texture preference is subjective; may not be comfortable for all users

6. Flavored Condoms

Flavored condoms are designed for oral sex, offering a variety of flavors to make the experience more enjoyable.

Benefits:

- Enhances the experience of oral sex
- Available in a wide range of flavors

Considerations:

- May contain sugars or flavorings that can cause irritation for some users
- Primarily intended for oral use; check compatibility for vaginal or anal use

7. Ultra-Thin Condoms

Ultra-thin condoms are designed to maximize sensitivity and provide a more natural feel during intercourse.

Benefits:

- Enhances sensitivity and pleasure
- Effective in preventing pregnancy and STIs

Considerations:

- Slightly higher risk of breakage compared to standard condoms
- Should be used with adequate lubrication to prevent tearing

★ **How to Use Condoms Correctly**

Using condoms correctly is crucial for their effectiveness in preventing pregnancy and STIs. Here is a step-by-step guide on how to use condoms properly:

Step 1 : Checking the Expiry Date

Always check the expiry date on the condom package. Expired condoms can be less effective and more prone to breakage.

Step 2 : Opening the Package

Carefully open the condom package to avoid tearing the condom. Do not use teeth or sharp objects.

Step 3 : Pinching the Tip

Pinch the tip of the condom to leave space for semen collection. This prevents the condom from bursting during ejaculation.

Step 4: Rolling It On

Place the condom on the head of the erect penis and roll it down to the base. Ensure it is rolled out completely and there are no air bubbles.

Step 5: During Intercourse

Ensure the condom stays in place during intercourse. If it slips off, stop and put on a new condom before continuing.

Step 6 :After Ejaculation

After ejaculation, hold the base of the condom while withdrawing to prevent it from slipping off. Carefully remove and dispose of the condom in the trash.

★   **Enhancing Pleasure with Condoms**

While some people believe condoms reduce sensitivity, there are various ways to enhance pleasure while using them.

1.   **Using Lubricants**

Lubricants can reduce friction and increase pleasure. Water-based and silicone-based lubricants are safe to use with most condoms. Apply a small amount inside the condom and more outside for maximum effect.

2. Experimenting with Different Types

Experiment with different types of condoms, such as textured or ultra-thin varieties, to find what enhances pleasure for you and your partner.

3. Warming Up

Engage in ample foreplay to ensure both partners are aroused before using the condom. This can enhance overall sexual satisfaction.

4. Incorporating Other Sex Toys

Incorporate sex toys, such as vibrators or cock rings, to enhance pleasure while using condoms. These toys can provide additional stimulation and variety.

5.Communicating with Your Partner

Open communication with your partner about what feels good can greatly enhance sexual pleasure. Discuss preferences and experiment together to find what works best.

★ **Addressing Common Concerns**

Understanding and addressing common concerns about condoms can help improve their acceptance and usage.

1.   Allergies

Latex allergies can cause discomfort or allergic reactions. If you or your partner are allergic to latex, opt for polyurethane or polyisoprene condoms.

2. Breakage

Condom breakage can occur due to improper usage or expired products. Ensure correct usage and check expiry dates to minimize this risk.

2. Reduced Sensitivity

While some people feel condoms reduce sensitivity, using ultra-thin condoms or applying lubricants can help enhance sensation.

Conclusion

Condoms are a crucial tool for safe and responsible sexual activity. By understanding the different types of condoms, how to use them correctly, and ways to enhance pleasure, individuals and couples can enjoy a satisfying and safe sexual experience. Open communication, proper usage, and experimentation with different condom types and lubricants can help maximize the benefits of condoms and contribute to a fulfilling sexual relationship.

Chapter

9

Chapter Outline

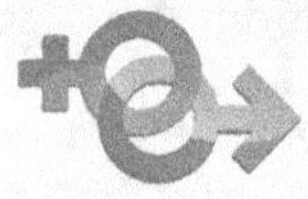

- Understanding oral sex
- Preparation of oral Sex
- Techniques of giving oral sex

- Specific technique of cunnilingus & fellatio
- Advance techniques
- Safety & precautions

Oral sex is a deeply intimate and pleasurable form of sexual activity that involves using the mouth, lips, and tongue to stimulate a partner's genitals. This chapter aims to provide a comprehensive guide to various techniques and tricks to ensure both partners find maximum satisfaction. It is crucial to approach oral sex with open communication, mutual consent, and a willingness to explore and understand each other's desires and boundaries.

★ **Understanding Oral Sex**

Oral sex encompasses a range of activities where the mouth is used to stimulate the genitals. For many, it is an integral part of foreplay and can also serve as a main sexual act. Its popularity stems from its ability to provide intense pleasure and intimacy.

Communication and Consent: Before engaging in oral sex, it's essential to have a candid conversation with your partner about boundaries, preferences, and any concerns. Consent is paramount, and both partners should feel comfortable and enthusiastic about the experience.

★ Preparation

Hygiene : Cleanliness is crucial for a pleasant oral sex experience. Both partners should ensure that they are clean and fresh. This can involve showering, brushing teeth, and using mouthwash beforehand.

Comfort : Creating a comfortable and relaxing environment can significantly enhance the experience. This could include soft lighting, comfortable bedding, and a private space free from interruptions.

Mental State : Being mentally prepared and relaxed is essential. Take the time to connect emotionally with your partner, ensuring that both of you are in the right frame of mind to enjoy the experience.

★ Techniques for Giving Oral Sex

Starting Slowly : Begin with gentle kisses and licks around the genital area. Building anticipation can heighten pleasure. Explore your partner's reactions and listen to their cues.

Use of Hands : Incorporate your hands to provide additional stimulation. For women, gently parting the labia or using fingers to stimulate the clitoris while licking can enhance pleasure. For men, using a hand to stroke the shaft while focusing oral attention on the head can be very effective.

Variety of Motions: Experiment with different movements. For example, swirling the tongue, alternating between sucking and licking, and using varying pressures can create a more dynamic experience.

Listening to Your Partner: Pay close attention to your partner's verbal and non-verbal cues. Adjust your technique based on their reactions. Moans, changes in breathing, and body movements can all provide valuable feedback.

Changing Speeds and Pressure: Don't be afraid to vary your speed and the intensity of your movements. Alternating between slow, sensual licks and faster, more intense motions can keep your partner on edge.

★   **Specific Techniques for Cunnilingus**

Exploring the Anatomy: Understanding the female anatomy is key. Focus on the clitoris, labia, and vaginal opening. Each area can provide different sensations.

Consistent Rhythm : Once you find a rhythm that your partner enjoys, try to maintain it. Consistency can help build towards a climax.

Using Different Parts of the Mouth : Incorporate your lips, tongue, and entire mouth for varied sensations. Lightly sucking the clitoris, followed by gentle flicks of the tongue, can be particularly stimulating.

Incorporating Moans and Sounds : The auditory aspect of sex can enhance the experience. Soft moans and verbal affirmations can increase arousal and provide positive feedback.

★   **Specific Techniques for Fellatio**

Understanding the Anatomy : Focus on the penis, paying particular attention to the head (glans) and the frenulum, which is the sensitive underside area where the shaft meets the head.

Incorporating Deep Throat Techniques : For those comfortable with it, deep throat techniques can provide intense pleasure. Start slowly and only go as deep as is comfortable. Practice can help improve your ability to take more of the penis into your mouth.

Hand and Mouth Coordination : Use your hand to stroke the base of the penis while your mouth focuses on the head and upper shaft. This combined stimulation can be highly effective.

Enhancing Pleasure with Temperature Play : Using warm or cold drinks beforehand can create interesting temperature contrasts. For example, sipping on warm tea or cold water and then using your mouth can heighten sensations.

★　　Advanced Techniques

Use of Toys : Introducing sex toys, such as vibrators, can add an extra layer of stimulation. Vibrators can be used on the clitoris during cunnilingus or on the perineum during fellatio to enhance pleasure.

Edging : Edging involves bringing your partner close to orgasm multiple times without allowing them to climax. This can build up a more intense final orgasm. Communicate clearly to avoid frustration and ensure it remains enjoyable.

Multi-Tasking : Combining oral sex with other forms of sexual stimulation, such as manual or penetrative play, can provide a fuller experience. For example, using a finger to stimulate the G-spot during cunnilingus or massaging the testicles during fellatio can be highly pleasurable.

Role Play and Fantasy : Exploring different scenarios and fantasies can heighten arousal. Discuss and agree upon any fantasies beforehand to ensure both partners are comfortable and willing participants.

★ Safety and Health Considerations

Protection : Using protection, such as dental dams or condoms, can prevent the transmission of sexually transmitted infections (STIs). It's important to prioritize safety, especially with new or multiple partners.

Regular Health Checks : Regular sexual health screenings are essential for maintaining overall health and well-being. Both partners should be aware of their STI status and communicate openly about it.

Respecting Limits : It's crucial to recognize and respect your partner's boundaries. Not all techniques or actions will be comfortable or enjoyable for everyone. Always prioritize mutual comfort and enjoyment.

Conclusion

Feedback and Communication : After engaging in oral sex, take the time to discuss what worked well and areas for improvement. This feedback can help both partners become more attuned to each other's needs and preferences.

Building Trust and Intimacy : Oral sex can significantly enhance intimacy and trust in a relationship. The act of giving and receiving pleasure in such a personal way can deepen the emotional connection between partners.

Continuous Learning : Sexual preferences and techniques can evolve over time. Encourage ongoing exploration and learning to keep the sexual relationship fulfilling and exciting.

Chapter
10

Chapter Outline

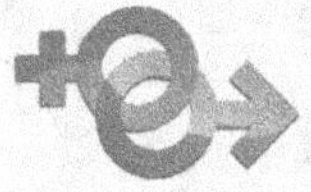

- Types of sexual excitement material
- Working of sexual excitement material

- Benifit of sex excitement material
- Aise effects of sex excitement material
- Choosing the right product

In the quest for enhanced sexual excitement, many people turn to various topical products designed to heighten sensitivity, increase pleasure, and create a more engaging sexual experience. This chapter focuses on the different types of sexual excitement materials, including creams, oils, gels, and other products. We will explore how they work, their benefits, potential side effects, and how to choose the right product for your needs.

Types of Sexual Excitement Materials

1. Arousal Creams and Gels

- **Function:** These products are designed to increase blood flow and sensitivity to the applied area, usually the genitals. They often contain ingredients like menthol, peppermint, or L-arginine, which create a tingling or warming sensation.

- **Benefits :** Arousal creams and gels can enhance sexual pleasure, making it easier to achieve orgasm or experience heightened arousal. For many people, these products serve as an effective way to intensify sexual experiences, whether used alone or with a partner.

- **Application :** Typically applied directly to the clitoris or penis before sexual activity, these products should be used according to the instructions provided. Some may require a few minutes to take effect, so planning ahead is beneficial.

Popular Ingredients :

- **Menthol:** Known for its cooling sensation, it stimulates nerve endings and increases sensitivity.
- **Peppermint Oil :** Provides a tingling effect that can enhance arousal.
- **L-Arginine : An** amino acid that increases nitric oxide levels, promoting blood flow and sensitivity.

2. Massage Oils

- **Function :** Massage oils are used to enhance foreplay and intimacy through sensual massage. They often contain essential oils known for their aphrodisiac properties, such as lavender, sandalwood, or ylang-ylang.

- **Benefits :** Massage oils promote relaxation, reduce stress, and increase physical intimacy, which can lead to greater sexual excitement. They can transform an ordinary massage into a deeply sensual experience, enhancing emotional connection and arousal.

- **Application :** Used during foreplay, massage oils are applied to the skin and massaged in with gentle, sensual strokes. The act of massaging not only relaxes the muscles but also builds anticipation and excitement.

Popular Ingredients :

- **Lavender :** Known for its calming properties, it can help reduce anxiety and set a relaxing mood.
- **Sandalwood :** An exotic scent that has been used for centuries as an aphrodisiac.
- **Ylang-Ylang :** Often used in aromatherapy to increase libido and reduce stress.

3. Lubricants

- **Function :** Lubricants reduce friction during sexual activity, making it more comfortable and pleasurable. Some lubricants are specifically formulated to enhance arousal with warming or cooling sensations.

- **Benefits :** Lubricants prevent discomfort and pain during sex, especially for individuals who experience vaginal dryness or for use during anal sex. Enhanced lubricants can add a new dimension to sexual experiences with their stimulating effects.

- **Application :** Applied to the genitals, sex toys, or condoms before and during sexual activity. It's important to choose the right type of lubricant based on the activity (water-based, silicone-based, or oil-based).

Types :

- **Water-Based Lubricants :** Versatile and safe to use with all sex toys and condoms.
- **Silicone-Based Lubricants :** Long-lasting and ideal for water activities, but not compatible with silicone toys.
- **Oil-Based Lubricants :** Provide a slippery feel but can degrade latex condoms and are harder to clean up.

4. Enhancement Sprays

- **Function** : Enhancement sprays are often used to prolong erection or delay ejaculation in men. They typically contain mild numbing agents like lidocaine or benzocaine.

- **Benefits** : They can help men maintain an erection longer, which can enhance sexual excitement and satisfaction for both partners. These sprays can be particularly useful for individuals experiencing premature ejaculation.

- **Application** : Sprayed directly onto the penis before sexual activity, with a brief waiting period to allow the numbing agent to take effect. It's important to follow the product's instructions to avoid over-application.

Popular Ingredients :

- **Lidocaine** : A local anesthetic that reduces sensitivity and helps delay ejaculation.
- **Benzocaine** : Another anesthetic commonly used in desensitizing sprays.

★ How Sexual Excitement Materials Work

These products work primarily through two mechanisms: increasing blood flow and altering sensation.

1. Increased Blood Flow

Many creams and gels contain vasodilators that help widen blood vessels, increasing blood flow to the applied area. This heightened blood flow can increase sensitivity and arousal. Ingredients like L-arginine work by boosting nitric oxide levels in the blood, which helps to dilate blood vessels and improve circulation.

2. Altered Sensation

Ingredients like menthol, peppermint, and capsaicin (found in chili peppers) can create warming, cooling, or tingling sensations. These sensations can enhance the physical experience and increase excitement by stimulating the nerve endings and heightening sensitivity in the applied area.

★ **Benefits of Sexual Excitement Materials**

1. **Enhanced Sensitivity :** By increasing blood flow and altering sensations, these products can make sexual experiences more intense and pleasurable. Users often report heightened sensations and a more profound sexual response.

2. **Improved Sexual Function :** For individuals facing challenges like vaginal dryness, erectile dysfunction, or delayed orgasm, these products can provide much-needed assistance. They can make sexual activity more comfortable and enjoyable, improving overall sexual function and satisfaction.

3. **Increased Intimacy :** Products like massage oils can help couples connect on a deeper level, fostering intimacy and enhancing overall sexual satisfaction. The act of giving and receiving a sensual massage can strengthen emotional bonds and increase arousal.

4. **Greater Variety :** Trying new products can add variety to a sexual relationship, keeping things exciting and preventing routine. Exploring different sensations and experiences can reignite passion and interest in long-term relationships.

★ Potential Side Effects

While these products can offer many benefits, they may also have potential side effects, including:

1. **Allergic Reactions :** Ingredients in some products can cause allergic reactions, such as itching, redness, or swelling. It's essential to perform a patch test before full application. Individuals with sensitive skin should be particularly cautious and choose hypoallergenic options.

2. **Sensitivity Issues :** Some individuals may find the sensations (tingling, warming, cooling) too intense or uncomfortable. It's important to start with a small amount and see how your body reacts before applying more.

3. **Interactions with Condoms :** Oil-based products can degrade latex condoms, making them less effective. It's important to choose condom-compatible products if you're using condoms for protection. Water-based or silicone-based lubricants are generally safe to use with condoms.

4. **Infections :** Improper use of these products, such as using them internally without proper hygiene, can increase the risk of infections. Always follow the product's instructions and maintain good hygiene practices.

★ Choosing the Right Product

When selecting a sexual excitement material, consider the following factors:

1. **Ingredients :** Look for products with high-quality, natural ingredients, and avoid those with potentially irritating chemicals or allergens. Reading the ingredient list and understanding what each component does can help you make an informed decision.

2. **Purpose :** Choose a product designed for your specific needs, whether it's enhancing arousal, providing lubrication, or increasing intimacy through massage. Different products cater to different aspects of sexual excitement, so it's important to identify your primary goal.

3. **Compatibility :** Ensure the product is compatible with any condoms or sex toys you plan to use. This is crucial to prevent damage to your toys or reducing the effectiveness of your condoms.

4. **Reviews and Recommendations :** Read reviews and seek recommendations from trusted sources to find reputable and effective products. User experiences can provide valuable insights into the effectiveness and safety of a product.

5. **Personal Preferences :** Consider your own and your partner's preferences regarding scents, textures, and sensations. What works for one person may not work for another, so personal experimentation can help you find the best product.

Conclusion

Sexual excitement materials, including creams, oils, gels, and sprays, offer a wide range of benefits for enhancing sexual pleasure and intimacy. By understanding how these products work and choosing the right one for your needs, you can enrich your sexual experiences and strengthen your intimate relationships. Always prioritize safety and comfort, and don't hesitate to experiment with different products to find what works best for you and your partner. With the right approach, these materials can play a significant role in achieving a fulfilling and exciting sexual life.

Chapter

11

 **Chapter Outline** 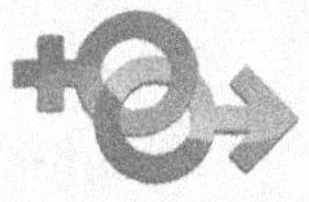

- Understanding anal anatomy
- Benifit of anal sex
- Preparation of anal sex
- Addressing common myths

- Techniques of anal sex
- Increasing pleasure of anal sex
- Safety & consent

Anal sex can be a source of immense pleasure for many individuals and couples. Despite being a topic often surrounded by myths and stigma, understanding and exploring anal sex can lead to satisfying and enjoyable experiences. This chapter aims to provide a detailed and comprehensive guide to anal sex, covering anatomy, preparation, techniques, safety, and tips for maximizing pleasure.

★ **Understanding Anal Anatomy**

To fully appreciate and enjoy anal sex, it's important to understand the anatomy involved:

- **Anus :** The external opening of the rectum. It is surrounded by sphincter muscles that control the passage of stool and can provide pleasurable sensations when stimulated.

- **Rectum :** The internal chamber connected to the anus, part of the digestive system. It can also be a source of pleasure when stimulated properly.

- **Prostate :** A gland in men located just inside the rectum, often referred to as the "male G-spot" or "P-spot." Stimulation of the prostate can lead to intense orgasms.

- **Nerve Endings :** The anus and surrounding area are rich in nerve endings, making it highly sensitive and capable of producing pleasurable sensations.

★ **Benefits of Anal Sex**

Engaging in anal sex can offer several benefits, including:

- **Enhanced Pleasure :** The anus and rectum have many nerve endings, making them highly sensitive to stimulation.

- **Prostate Stimulation** : For men, anal sex can stimulate the prostate, potentially leading to powerful orgasms.

- **Variety and Novelty :** Incorporating anal play into your sex life can add variety and keep things exciting.

- **Deeper Intimacy :** Trust and communication required for anal sex can deepen the emotional bond between partners.

★ **Preparation for Anal Sex**

Proper preparation is crucial for a pleasurable and safe anal sex experience:

1. Communication

- **Discuss Boundaries :** Talk openly with your partner about your desires, boundaries, and any concerns.

- **Set Expectations :** Agree on what you both want to try and establish a safe word for stopping if needed.

2. Hygiene

- **Cleaning :** Thoroughly clean the anal area before engaging in anal sex. Some people choose to use an enema, but it's not always necessary.

- **Short Nails :** Ensure fingernails are trimmed and clean to avoid scratching sensitive tissues.

3. Lubrication

- **Use Plenty :** The anus does not produce natural lubrication, so a generous amount of lubricant is essential.
- **Type of Lubricant :** Use a high-quality water-based or silicone-based lubricant. Avoid oil-based lubricants with latex condoms as they can cause breakage.

4. Relaxation

- **Take It Slow :** Start with plenty of foreplay to relax and arouse both partners.

- **Breathing Techniques :** Practice deep breathing to help relax the anal muscles.

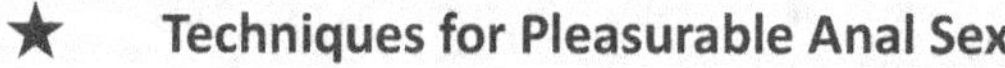 **Techniques for Pleasurable Anal Sex**

1. Foreplay and Warm-Up

- **Start Small :** Begin with external stimulation using fingers, a small anal toy, or a butt plug.

- **Gentle Massage :** Use your fingers to gently massage the anus and surrounding area.

2. Insertion

- **Go Slow :** Slowly and gently insert a well-lubricated finger or toy, allowing the muscles to relax and adjust.

- **Communicate :** Check in with your partner frequently to ensure they are comfortable and relaxed.

3. Positions

- **Doggy Style :** Allows for deep penetration and easy access to the anus.
- **Spooning :** Provides a more intimate and controlled angle of penetration.
- **Missionary :** The receiving partner on their back with legs raised, allowing for good control and communication.

4. Prostate Stimulation

- **Finding the Prostate :** For men, the prostate can be stimulated by curling a finger or toy towards the front of the body.
- **Techniques :** Gentle pressure and massaging movements can lead to intense pleasure and even prostate orgasms.

★ Enhancing Pleasure

1. Incorporate Toys

- **Butt Plugs :** Use butt plugs to help relax the anal muscles and enhance arousal.

- **Prostate Massagers :** For men, prostate massagers can provide targeted stimulation.

- **Vibrating Toys :** Add extra sensations with vibrating anal toys.

O2. Combine with Other Stimulation

- **Oral and Manual Stimulation :** Combine anal play with oral sex or manual stimulation of the genitals for enhanced pleasure.
- **Double Penetration :** For those interested, using a dildo or vibrator vaginally while being penetrated anally can intensify sensations.

3. Focus on Relaxation and Arousal

- **Patience :** Take your time and don't rush the experience.
- **Build Up Slowly :** Gradually increase the intensity and depth of penetration as comfort and arousal increase.

★ **Safety and Consent**

1. Use Protection

- **Condoms :** Use condoms to reduce the risk of sexually transmitted infections (STIs) and make cleanup easier.
- **Change Condoms :** If switching between vaginal and anal sex, use a new condom to avoid transferring bacteria.

2. Listen to Your Body

- **Pain is a Signal :** If you or your partner experience pain, stop and communicate. Pain indicates something isn't right.
- **Take Breaks :** Take breaks if needed to relax and adjust.

3. Aftercare

- **Clean Up :** Clean the anal area and any toys used with warm water and soap.
- **Comfort :** Spend time cuddling and reassuring each other after the experience to enhance emotional intimacy.

★ **Addressing Common Myths and Concerns**

1. Myth: Anal Sex is Always Painful

- **Truth :** With proper preparation, communication, and relaxation, anal sex can be pleasurable and pain-free.

2. Myth: Only Gay Men Enjoy Anal Sex

- **Truth :** People of all sexual orientations and genders can enjoy anal sex.

3. Myth: Anal Sex is Dirty

- **Truth :** Proper hygiene can make anal sex a clean and enjoyable experience.

4. Concern: Fear of Injury

- **Solution :** Use plenty of lubricant, go slow, and communicate. Start with smaller toys or fingers and gradually progress.

Conclusion

Exploring anal sex can open up new realms of pleasure and intimacy for you and your partner. By understanding the anatomy, preparing properly, using the right techniques, and prioritizing safety and communication, you can create a positive and enjoyable anal sex experience. Remember, the key to pleasurable anal sex is patience, relaxation, and mutual respect. Enjoy the journey of discovery and deepen your connection with your partner through this shared exploration.

Chapter 12

Chapter Outline

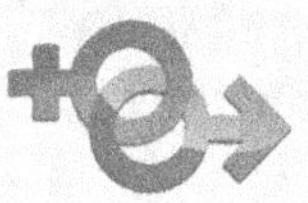

- Physiological consideration
- Psychological & emotional factors
- Related Dynamics
- Practical tips for optimal timing

Sexual satisfaction is a fundamental component of a healthy relationship. It fosters intimacy, strengthens emotional bonds, and contributes to overall well-being. One factor that can significantly influence sexual satisfaction is timing. Understanding how timing affects sexual encounters can help partners enhance their experiences and meet each other's needs more effectively. This chapter explores whether sex timing matters in satisfying your partner, delving into physiological, psychological, and relational aspects.

★ Physiological Considerations

1.Circadian Rhythms and Hormonal Fluctuations

Our bodies follow a circadian rhythm, a natural 24-hour cycle that affects various biological processes, including sexual desire and performance. Hormone levels, particularly testosterone, vary throughout the day, influencing libido and arousal.

Morning: Testosterone levels peak in the morning, which can enhance sexual desire and arousal. Morning sex can be particularly satisfying due to higher energy levels and increased sensitivity.

Evening: While testosterone levels might be lower, evening sex offers the benefit of relaxation and winding down. The release of oxytocin during sex can promote feelings of closeness and relaxation, making evening an ideal time for many couples.

2. Menstrual Cycle Phases

For women, the menstrual cycle can significantly impact sexual desire and satisfaction. Understanding these phases can help in timing sexual activity to enhance pleasure.

- **Follicular Phase:** This phase starts on the first day of menstruation and lasts until ovulation. Sexual desire often increases as ovulation approaches due to rising estrogen levels.

- **Ovulation:** Occurring around the midpoint of the cycle, ovulation is marked by a peak in libido driven by a surge in hormones. This is often the best time for sexual satisfaction.

- **Luteal Phase:** Following ovulation, progesterone levels rise, which can sometimes dampen sexual desire. Awareness of this phase can help partners adjust their expectations and find other ways to maintain intimacy.

★ Psychological and Emotional Factors

1. Stress Levels and Mental State

Stress and mental state significantly impact sexual satisfaction. Choosing the right time for intimacy can enhance the overall experience by ensuring both partners are relaxed and emotionally available.

- **Stress Reduction:** Engaging in sexual activity during low-stress periods, such as weekends or after a relaxing activity, can improve satisfaction.

- **Emotional Readiness:** Both partners should be in a good mental state, free from significant distractions or worries. This can lead to a deeper emotional connection and a more fulfilling experience.

2. Emotional Connection and Bonding

The emotional connection between partners plays a crucial role in sexual satisfaction. Timing sex to align with moments of strong emotional bonding can enhance the experience.

- **Quality Time:** Scheduling sex after spending quality time together, such as after a date night or a shared hobby, can strengthen the emotional connection.

- **Communication:** Open and honest communication about desires, needs, and preferences can help in timing sex to maximize satisfaction.

★ Relational Dynamics

1. Synchronizing Desires

Mismatched sexual desires can be a common issue in relationships. Finding a balance that satisfies both partners requires understanding and compromise.

- **Negotiation and Compromise:** Partners can discuss their preferred times and frequencies for sex, finding a schedule that works for both. Regular, planned intimacy can help maintain a healthy sexual relationship.

- **Spontaneity:** While planning is important, spontaneity also plays a crucial role. Unexpected moments of intimacy can add excitement and novelty to the relationship.

2. Life Stages and Responsibilities

Different life stages and responsibilities can affect the timing and frequency of sexual activity. Adjusting to these changes is essential for maintaining sexual satisfaction.

- **Young Adults:** Typically have more flexibility and energy for frequent sexual activity. Spontaneity is easier to manage, and both partners may be more open to exploring different times for intimacy.
- **Parents:** With children and demanding schedules, timing sex can become more challenging. Finding moments when both partners are free from distractions and responsibilities is key.
- **Older Adults:** Changes in sexual function and desire can occur with aging. Open communication and flexibility in timing can help adapt to these changes and maintain satisfaction.

★ Practical Tips for Optimal Timing

1. Prioritizing Intimacy

Making intimacy a priority, despite busy schedules, can significantly enhance sexual satisfaction. Setting aside dedicated time for sex ensures that both partners feel valued and connected.

2. Healthy Lifestyle Choices

Maintaining a healthy lifestyle with regular exercise, balanced nutrition, and adequate sleep can positively impact sexual desire and performance. This, in turn, makes finding the right time for sex more rewarding.

3. Adapting to Changes

Life circumstances and personal preferences can change. Being flexible and willing to adapt to new situations can help maintain a fulfilling sexual relationship.

4. Open Communication

Continuous, open communication about sexual needs and preferences is fundamental. Partners should feel comfortable discussing what times work best for them and be willing to make adjustments.

Conclusion

Timing indeed matters in sexual satisfaction, influencing physiological readiness, emotional connection, and relational harmony. By understanding the importance of timing and considering the unique needs and preferences of both partners, couples can enhance their sexual experiences and deepen their emotional bonds.

Chapter Outline

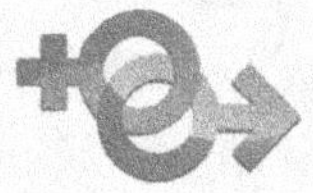

- Fundamentals of oral sex
- How to perform cunnilingus (pussy licking)
- How to perform anilingus (Licking anus)
- How to perform fallatio (blowjob)

Oral sex is a highly intimate act that can bring immense pleasure to both partners when performed correctly and consensually. This chapter will delve into the techniques and best practices for performing cunnilingus (licking the vulva), anilingus (licking the anus), and fellatio (blowjob), ensuring maximum comfort and pleasure.

The Foundation of Oral Sex: Consent and Communication
Before engaging in any sexual activity, it is crucial to establish clear consent and open communication with your partner. Discussing boundaries, preferences, and comfort levels helps ensure a positive and enjoyable experience for both parties.

- Understanding Consent: Consent must be enthusiastic, ongoing, and can be withdrawn at any time.

- Effective Communication: Talk about likes, dislikes, and any concerns to create a safe and pleasurable environment.

nfluencing physiological readiness, emotional connection, and relational harmony. By understanding the importance of timing and considering the unique needs and preferences of both partners, couples can enhance their sexual experiences and deepen their emotional bonds.

★ <u>How to Perform Cunnilingus (Licking Pussy)</u>

Understanding Female Anatomy:

- The vulva includes the outer and inner labia, the clitoris, and the vaginal opening.
- The clitoris, with over 8,000 nerve endings, is highly sensitive and often the focal point for pleasure.

Techniques and Tips:

- **1. Preparation and Hygiene:**

    - Ensure both partners are clean and comfortable.
    - Use a comfortable position where both can relax, such as lying down or sitting on the edge of the bed.

- **2. Starting Slow:**

    - Begin with gentle kissing and licking around the thighs and outer labia.
    - Gradually work towards the inner labia and clitoris to build anticipation and arousal.

- **3. Clitoral Stimulation:**

    - Use the tip of your tongue to make small, circular motions around the clitoris.
    - Vary the pressure and speed based on your partner's responses .

- Incorporate light sucking on the clitoris for added stimulation.

- 4. Exploring the Vulva:

  - Use your tongue to explore the entire vulva, including the inner labia and vaginal opening.

  - Gentle, rhythmic licking can enhance pleasure and arousal.

- Communication and Feedback:

  - Encourage your partner to guide you on what feels best.

  - Pay attention to verbal and non-verbal cues to adjust your technique accordingly.

- **6. Incorporating Fingers:**

  - Combine oral stimulation with gentle insertion of fingers into the vagina.

  - Use a "come-hither" motion to stimulate the G-spot while continuing oral stimulation on the clitoris.

- ★ **<u>How to Perform Anilingus (Licking Anus)</u>**

- **Understanding Anilingus:**

  - Anilingus involves stimulating the anus with the mouth, lips, and tongue. It can be highly pleasurable when performed with care and consent.

- **Techniques and Tips:**

    - **1. Preparation and Hygiene:**

    - Cleanliness is paramount. Both partners should shower and clean the anal area thoroughly.
    - Consider using dental dams for added protection.

    - **2. Starting Slow:**

    - Begin with gentle kisses and licks around the buttocks and perineum (the area between the genitals and anus).
    - Gradually move closer to the anus, increasing the intensity of stimulation.

- **3. Techniques for Stimulation:**

    - Use the tip of your tongue to make gentle, circular motions around the anus.
    - Lightly flick or press the tongue against the anal opening.
    - Incorporate gentle suction and rhythmic licking for added pleasure.

- **4. Comfort and Communication:**

    - Ensure your partner is comfortable and relaxed.
    - Maintain open communication to gauge comfort levels and adjust techniques as needed.

★ <u>How to Perform Fellatio (Blowjob)</u>

- **Understanding Male Anatomy:**

  - The penis consists of the shaft, glans (head), and frenulum (the sensitive area just below the glans).
  - The testicles are also sensitive and can be included in stimulation.

Techniques and Tips:

1. Preparation and Comfort:

- Ensure both partners are clean and comfortable.
- Use a position that allows easy access and comfort, such as lying down or sitting.

2. Starting Slow:

- Begin with gentle kissing and licking around the thighs and base of the penis.
- Gradually move to the shaft and glans, increasing the intensity of stimulation

3. Techniques for Stimulation:

- Use your tongue to make swirling motions around the glans and frenulum.
- Vary the speed and pressure of your movements, incorporating gentle suction.
- Take the penis into your mouth, creating a seal with your lips and using a rhythmic bobbing motion.

4. Incorporating Hands:

- Use your hands to stroke the shaft while your mouth focuses on the glans.
- Combine different techniques, such as twisting and squeezing gently, to enhance pleasure.

5. Communication and Feedback

- Encourage your partner to guide you on what feels best.
- Pay attention to verbal and non-verbal cues to adjust your technique accordingly.

6. Stimulation of the Testicles

- Gently caress and fondle the testicles with your hands or mouth.
- Be gentle and attentive to your partner's comfort levels.

7. Safe Sex Practices

- Importance of Protection: Using protection, such as condoms and dental dams, reduces the risk of sexually transmitted infections (STIs) and enhances safety.

8. Use of Condoms and Dental Dams:

- **Condoms:** Can be used during fellatio to reduce STI risk.
- **Dental Dams:** Thin sheets of latex or polyurethane that provide a barrier during cunnilingus and anilingus .

9. Hygiene and Cleanliness: Maintaining cleanliness before and after sexual activity is crucial for health and comfort. Washing hands and genital areas can prevent infections and enhance the experience.

Conclusion

Oral sex can be an intensely pleasurable experience when performed with care, consent, and open communication. By understanding your partner's anatomy, using various techniques, and prioritizing hygiene and safety, you can enhance intimacy and satisfaction for both partners. Continual learning and open discussions about preferences and boundaries will lead to deeper intimacy and enjoyment .

Chapter Outline

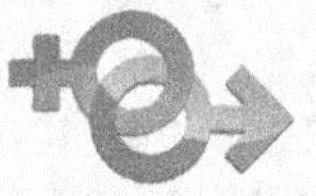

- ❏ Understanding distance sex
- ❏ Establishing consent & boundaries
- ❏ Privacy & security

- ❏ Techniques & activities
- ❏ Communicating & feedback
- ❏ After care

In today's interconnected world, distance sex, also known as mobile sex or virtual intimacy, has become increasingly prevalent. This chapter explores how technology facilitates intimate connections between partners who are physically separated. It examines the benefits, challenges, techniques, and ethical considerations associated with engaging in sexual activities through digital means.

★ Understanding Distance Sex

- **Definition and Evolution:** Distance sex encompasses a range of activities where partners use technology to engage in sexual interactions despite being apart. It includes video calls, messaging, virtual reality (VR), and remote-controlled sex toys.

- **Technological Facilitators:**
    - ○ **Video Calls:** Platforms like Zoom, Skype, FaceTime, and specialized adult platforms allow partners to see and hear each other in real-time, enhancing intimacy.

- **Messaging Apps:** Texting, sexting, and sending intimate messages or media build anticipation and connection.

- **Virtual Reality (VR):** Emerging technologies offer immersive experiences where partners can interact in virtual environments, enhancing sensory engagement.

★ **Establishing Consent and Boundaries**

- **Importance of Consent:** In distance sex, just as in physical intimacy, consent is paramount. Clear communication about boundaries, preferences, and comfort levels is crucial before engaging in any sexual activities.

- **Respecting Privacy and Security:**

  - **Privacy Concerns:** Discuss and agree on the use and storage of intimate content to protect both partners' privacy.
  - **Security Measures:** Use secure platforms and apps to minimize the risk of data breaches or unauthorized access to sensitive information.

★ **Techniques and Activities**

- **Building Anticipation:**
  - **Sexting and Messaging:** Use descriptive language, emojis, photos, or videos to create erotic tension and anticipation.
  - **Voice and Video Calls:** Engage in erotic conversations, share fantasies, or perform virtual stripteases to stimulate arousal.
  - **Mutual Masturbation:** Simultaneously pleasure yourselves while watching each other via video call, fostering intimacy and shared pleasure.

- **Enhancing Sensation:**
  - **Incorporating Sex Toys:**Utilize remote-controlled toys that can be synchronized over the internet for mutual pleasure and enhanced sensation.
  - **Virtual Reality (VR) Experiences:**Explore VR environments designed for sexual interaction, offering immersive sensory experiences and exploration of fantasies.

★ **Communication and Feedback**

Real-Time Interaction:

- **Verbal Guidance:**Guide each other with verbal cues and instructions during activities to enhance mutual satisfaction.
- **Non-Verbal Cues:** Pay attention to body language and reactions to adjust techniques and pace, ensuring a pleasurable experience for both partners.

★ **Privacy and Security Considerations**

Protecting Personal Information:

- **Choosing Secure Platforms:**Select reputable and secure apps or platforms for communication and content sharing.
- **Content Sharing Awareness:** Be mindful of the risks associated with sharing intimate content online and take steps to protect privacy and prevent unauthorized access.

★ **Aftercare and Emotional Connection**

Emotional Support and Connection:

- **Post-Session Communication:**Discuss feelings, experiences, and emotions to maintain emotional intimacy and connection.

- **Affection and Reassurance:**Provide emotional support and reassurance to each other after intimate sessions to strengthen the bond.

Conclusion

Distance sex offers a modern approach to maintaining intimacy and connection with a partner, overcoming physical barriers through technology. By prioritizing consent, privacy, and mutual satisfaction, couples can explore and enjoy fulfilling sexual experiences from afar. Open communication, respect for boundaries, and ongoing emotional connection are essential for creating a positive and enriching distance sex experience.

Chapter
15

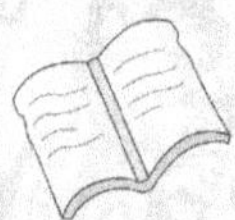 **Chapter Outline** 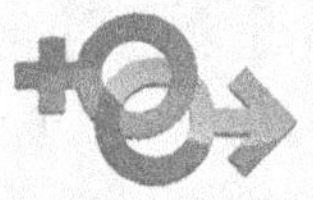

- Male erogenous zones
- Female erogenous zones
- Techniques for enhancing pleasure

Erogenous zones are areas of the body that are particularly sensitive to sexual stimulation and can contribute to sexual arousal and pleasure. Understanding these zones in both males and females can enhance intimate experiences and improve communication between partners.

★ Male Erogenous Zones

- **Penis:**The primary male sexual organ, consisting of the shaft, glans (head), and frenulum. It is highly sensitive to touch, especially the glans and frenulum.

  Techniques: Stroking, kissing, sucking, and varying pressure can stimulate different parts of the penis.

- **Scrotum:**The sac containing the testicles.

  Techniques: Light touching, gentle massaging, and kissing can enhance arousal.

- **Perineum** : The area between the scrotum and anus.

  Techniques: Light stroking or pressing can stimulate nerve endings and enhance arousal.

- **Anus**

  Techniques: Some men find gentle stimulation around the anus pleasurable, including light touching or massage.

- **Nipples**

  Techniques: Light touching, kissing, licking, and gentle biting can stimulate the nipples and enhance arousal.

- **Ears and Neck**

  Techniques:Gentle kissing, nibbling, and whispering can be highly arousing.

- **Other Areas**

  Some men may find other areas, such as the inner thighs, back of the knees, or feet, sensitive to sexual stimulation.

★ **Female Erogenous Zones**

- **Clitoris** : The clitoris is the most sensitive female erogenous zone, located above the vaginal opening.

  Techniques: Gentle circular motions, licking, and sucking can stimulate the clitoris and induce arousal.

  Clitoral Hood: Protects the clitoris and can also be sensitive to touch.

- **G-spot :** Located inside the vagina on the front wall, about 1-2 inches in.

  Techniques: Firm, rhythmic pressure with fingers or a curved sex toy can stimulate the G-spot and lead to intense pleasure.

- **Vagina**

  Techniques: Penetration, either with fingers, a penis, or a sex toy, can stimulate nerve endings within the vaginal walls.

- **Labia**

  Techniques: Light touching, kissing, and gentle pulling can stimulate the outer and inner labia.

- **Breasts and Nipples**

  Techniques: Kissing, licking, gentle biting, and caressing can stimulate the breasts and nipples.

  Areola: The darker area surrounding the nipple can also be sensitive to touch.

- **Anus**

  Techniques: Some women may find gentle stimulation around the anus pleasurable, including light touching or massage.

- **Ears and Neck**

  Techniques: Gentle kissing, nibbling, and soft blowing can be highly arousing.

Other Areas : Some women may find other areas, such as the inner thighs, back of the knees, or feet, sensitive to sexual stimulation.

3. Techniques for Enhancing Pleasure

- **Communication:** Openly discuss preferences, boundaries, and techniques with your partner to ensure mutual satisfaction.

- **Foreplay :** Spend ample time on foreplay to build arousal and anticipation, focusing on erogenous zones.

- **Experimentation :** Explore different techniques, pressures, and speeds to discover what feels best for both partners.

- **Incorporating Toys :** Use sex toys designed for specific erogenous zones to enhance stimulation and pleasure.

- **Emotional Connection :** Building emotional intimacy outside of sexual encounters can deepen pleasure and satisfaction during intimacy.

- **Cultural and Personal Variations :** Erogenous zones and preferences can vary based on cultural backgrounds, personal experiences, and individual anatomy.

Conclusion

Understanding and exploring sexual erogenous zones in males and females can enhance sexual satisfaction and intimacy between partners. By communicating openly, experimenting with techniques, and focusing on mutual pleasure, couples can create fulfilling and enjoyable sexual experiences .

Acknowledgement

Writing "SeXDucation: Key to Satisfy" has been an enlightening journey, and I am deeply grateful to those who supported and inspired me along the way.

First and foremost, I want to thank my family and friends for their unwavering encouragement and understanding during this project. Your belief in me and my work has been a constant source of motivation.

I extend my heartfelt gratitude to the experts and colleagues who generously shared their insights and knowledge, enriching the content of this book. Your contributions have been invaluable.

Finally, I am profoundly thankful to my readers. Your curiosity and desire to explore and understand the intricacies of sexual relationships are the driving force behind this book. I hope "SeXDucation: Key to Satisfy" provides you with valuable insights and tools to enhance your relationships.

With profound gratitude,

Jeet Ghosh

www.ingramcontent.com/pod-product-compliance
Lightning Source LLC
Chambersburg PA
CBHW070743250726
48662CB00004B/1625